A Doula's Guide to Improving
Maternal Health for BIPOC Women

of related interest

Supporting Autistic People Through Pregnancy and Childbirth
Hayley Morgan, Emma Durman and Karen Henry
Forewords by Carly Jones, Wenn B. Lawson, and Sheena Byrom
ISBN 978 1 83997 105 1
eISBN 978 1 83997 106 8

My Black Motherhood
Mental Health, Stigma, Racism and the System
Sandra Igwe
ISBN 978 1 83997 008 5
eISBN 978 1 83997 009 2

Supporting Survivors of Sexual Abuse Through Pregnancy and Childbirth
A Guide for Midwives, Doulas and Other Healthcare Professionals
Kicki Hansard
Forewords by Penny Simkin and Phyllis Klaus
ISBN 978 1 84819 424 3
eISBN 978 0 85701 377 4

Women's Health Aromatherapy
A Clinically Evidence-Based Guide for Nurses, Midwives, Doulas and Therapists
Pam Conrad
ISBN 978 1 84819 425 0
eISBN 978 0 85701 378 1

Supporting Queer Birth
A Book for Birth Professionals and Parents
AJ Silver
ISBN 978 1 83997 045 0
eISBN 978 1 83997 046 7

Supporting Fat Birth
A Book for Birth Professionals and Parents
AJ Silver
ISBN 978 1 83997 633 9
eISBN 978 1 83997 634 6

A DOULA'S GUIDE TO
Improving Maternal Health for BIPOC Women

Jacquelyn Clemmons

Foreword by Desirée L. Israel

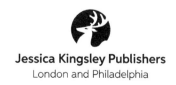

Jessica Kingsley Publishers
London and Philadelphia

First published in Great Britain in 2025 by Jessica Kingsley Publishers
An imprint of John Murray Press

2

Copyright © Jacquelyn Clemmons 2025
Foreword copyright © Desirée L. Israel 2025

The right of Jacquelyn Clemmons to be identified as the Author of the Work has been
asserted by her in accordance with the Copyright, Designs and Patents Act 1988.

Front cover image source: iStockphoto®. The cover image is for
illustrative purposes only, and any person featuring is a model.

A CIP catalogue record for this title is available from the
British Library and the Library of Congress

ISBN 978 1 83997 176 1
eISBN 978 1 83997 177 8

Printed and bound by CPI Group (UK) Ltd, Croydon, CR0 4YY

Jessica Kingsley Publishers' policy is to use papers that are natural,
renewable and recyclable products and made from wood grown in
sustainable forests. The logging and manufacturing processes are expected
to conform to the environmental regulations of the country of origin.

Jessica Kingsley Publishers
Carmelite House
50 Victoria Embankment
London EC4Y 0DZ

www.jkp.com

John Murray Press
Part of Hodder & Stoughton Ltd
An Hachette Company

Contents

Foreword

It is with immense joy and honor that I introduce you to *A Doula's Guide to Improving Maternal Health for BIPOC Women* by the extraordinary Jacquelyn Clemmons. This book is more than just a guide; it's a profound journey into the heart and soul of birth work, a heartfelt call to action, and a testament to the transformative power of self-development and genuine connection.

I've had the privilege of knowing Jacquelyn for over a decade, and our shared passion for the traditional ways of birthkeeping brought us together. We discovered a profound truth in our conversations—that everything in the realm of birth and postpartum support is interconnected. It encompasses not just the physical aspects but the mind, the spirit, and the dynamics of the family unit. This revelation laid the foundation for what you're about to embark on: a remarkable journey of self-discovery, empathy, and unwavering commitment to the well-being of BIPOC women during one of the most significant chapters of their lives.

Jacquelyn Clemmons is not just an author; she is a doula with a heart full of compassion and a spirit deeply rooted in the communities she serves. Her dedication to improving maternal health for BIPOC women is not merely professional—it's personal. This book is a testament to her lived experience, her wisdom, and her unwavering commitment to dismantling the barriers that disproportionately affect women of color during pregnancy and childbirth.

As a reproductive psychotherapist, trained birth and postpartum doula, herbalist, and certified breastfeeding specialist, I have had the privilege of supporting families across the full spectrum of reproductive experiences for over a decade. It was through this work that I learned the vital lesson that Jacquelyn's book emphasizes: to be truly effective in helping families, we must first check our egos at the door. We must recognize that the birth experience is not about us; it's about the birthing person and their journey. It's about acknowledging their unique circumstances, their fears and their hopes, and providing unwavering support, free from judgment or personal agenda.

In *A Doula's Guide to Improving Maternal Health for BIPOC Women*, Jacquelyn brilliantly highlights the critical importance of self-development. She invites all birth workers, whether seasoned veterans or those just starting their journey, to engage in introspection and growth. As we navigate the intricate web of birth work, it's essential to remember that we are not static beings. We are on a constant journey of growth and self-discovery, and the more we nurture our own development, the better equipped we become to support others.

The themes of self-development, rest, and ego-checking resonate deeply with me because they are the pillars upon which effective birth work is built. Jacquelyn's wisdom reminds us that true selflessness and genuine connection are the cornerstones of our practice. Birth workers: as you delve into these pages, be prepared to challenge your assumptions, question your biases, and emerge as even more compassionate, understanding, and empathetic advocates for the women and families you serve.

Connection and interdependence are at the core of this book, and they are the driving force behind effective birth work. Jacquelyn's insights remind us that every birthing experience is unique and sacred, and we must honor the diversity of traditions, beliefs, and perspectives that our clients bring to the table. In doing so, we create an environment where trust and collaboration can flourish, ultimately leading to better outcomes for the mothers and babies we serve.

As I reflect on the profound impact that birth work has had on my life and the lives of countless others, I am reminded of the words of

Maya Angelou: "We are more alike, my friends, than we are unalike." In the journey ahead, let us remember that we are all interconnected, and through our work, we have the power to uplift, empower, and transform lives.

Jacquelyn Clemmons's *A Doula's Guide to Improving Maternal Health for BIPOC Women* is not just a book; it's a guiding light for birth workers on their path toward more profound self-discovery, authentic connection, and transformative service. I am deeply honored to write this foreword and to witness the positive impact this book will undoubtedly have on birth workers and the communities they serve.

So, dear reader, I invite you to embark on this inspiring journey with an open heart and an eager spirit. Let Jacquelyn's words be your guide as you navigate the intricate and beautiful tapestry of maternal health, birth, and postpartum support. May you find inspiration, reflection, and renewed purpose within these pages.

In the pages that follow, you will discover the heart and soul of birth work—a world where empathy, connection, and selflessness reign supreme. May this book serve as a beacon of light and a source of inspiration on your journey to becoming the compassionate, skilled, and truly impactful doula that every birthing person deserves.

With gratitude and anticipation,
Desirée L. Israel, PhDc, LCSW-C, LICSW, LCSW, CBS

Special Dedications

First, I must give thanks to Abba. This has been quite a journey in publishing and writing this book. I have gone through many things in my life, and without being held together in my mind, body, and spirit, I would not have been able to complete this book.

To my children, my three little beans—my two daughters, Cherie-Amor and Dela Eden, and my son, Malachi. I have lived this thing out, being your mother, being pregnant with you, giving birth to you, experiencing life through you and with you. Much of my perspectives, moments, lessons, and curiosity would not have happened had you not been in my life.

I want to dedicate this book to my great-grandmother, Naomi Leslie. She was a grand midwife in North Carolina. I don't know how she got into this work, but to think that I even had it epigenetically in my DNA to do this line of work is remarkable. She's the earliest person I know in my lineage who has been involved in birth work.

I also want to dedicate this book to my grandmother, Flora, for always telling me the stories of my family and my elders and keeping our history alive. She always shared these stories with me in love. Grandma Flora always thought that nothing was impossible for me. Writing this book is something I would not have thought possible, but I can still hear her voice telling me, "Go ahead. I've got your back. I'm here. I've got your back." And those words of encouragement and her posture have allowed me to achieve many things in this world.

And my mother, Wanda. Watching you serve and love on the

geriatric population and the poor population my entire life impacted me greatly. I've watched you serve people who could not afford anything and who did not have much. Your heart has always leaned toward helping and serving people who could not otherwise receive care. And to see you serve them with a high level of excellence with medical care was a beautiful portrait of love. You have led with empathy and embraced others that were not receiving care in other spaces. You treat everyone with gentleness, respect, kindness, and the honor they deserve as human beings. You are an impeccable example of how to treat people with dignity. Whether they are homeless or not, you treat everyone the same. Your example has been a gift, that I've been blessed to witness my entire life.

I also want to thank my amazing husband, Hassan. The homey, lover, and friend God knew I needed. Thank you for being my rock, being there for me and supporting me, especially in moments where I don't know what else to do. You have been an amazing refreshing to my soul and I love you dearly.

Finally, I want to dedicate this book to my baby sister Victoria, whose life was taken in May of 2022. She was unfortunately a victim of postpartum homicide. Her life was taken shortly after giving birth to her son by her estranged husband. When I think about all the families and the women I have been able to serve over the years, it's the blessing to have served my family that resonates the most. Being able to serve my sister after she gave birth, and help talk her through breastfeeding was the last gift I was able to offer her. It was a blessing, but I know there's a part of me that still feels like I could have done more because I've been able to do so much more for other people. I want to dedicate this book to her justice and in honor of those forgotten women that are in domestic violence situations. They're not just pregnant, they're also dealing with heavy burdens people have no idea about. I can't imagine the burden of bringing in new life and trying to figure out how to preserve your own life. And so, I want to dedicate this book in love to her memory.

Introduction

One of the major issues I see in the birthing community right now is the centering of everyone but the person giving birth, regardless of their race. In the medical community, there is a desire to show up as an expert, whether it's the nurse, doctor, tech, doula, or midwife. While some of their expertize may be true, it is important to recognize that the person giving birth has their own expertize and experience. We should not be the center of someone else's birth experience at any point, and this issue extends even to doulas. We are not here to save the day.

In Western culture, there is a pervasive attitude that wants to center everyone but the person being served, and it is a problem. Therefore, I hope to shed light on the importance of personal development and self-focus. By developing ourselves personally, we can step outside the center of any particular situation, including serving people who are giving birth. It is crucial to be emotionally intelligent and aware enough to consider the stories and needs of others, serving them at the highest level possible. This requires us to acquire information, use tools, and maintain curiosity about people and the world around us.

However, it is equally important to ensure that we do not compromise our own boundaries or burn out. Birth workers are essential, but we need to be whole and continue to grow while taking care of ourselves—mind, body, and spirit. In other words, we need to become better so that we can serve better; because if any of these aspects are lacking, we are at a deficit. My hope is that each reader will reflect on themselves, their why, and approach this work authentically and honestly. Not everyone has to be a birth doula or postpartum doula; there are various roles within this field such as legislation, placenta encapsulation, childbirth education, or lactation support. It is crucial to be true to oneself and not pursue something that doesn't align with our personality or values. Doing so would only do a disservice to those we come into contact with.

As a woman of Black and indigenous heritage, I have had the privilege of working with women from various cultural backgrounds, including Caucasian, Latina, Asian, African American, African, and Caribbean women, for over 20 years. However, the depth of our connections does not solely rely on our shared racial or ethnic identities. It is the principles outlined in this book, which emphasize personal growth, understanding, and empathy, that have facilitated meaningful exchanges between us.

By the end of this book, my aim is for readers to assess where they truly stand on this journey and make the best decision for themselves on how they want to pursue this work. They should consider their ability and capacity to serve the people they want to serve, and then pursue that path with their mind, body, and spirit. If more people approach birth work in this way, the ripple effect will be profound. We will find our tribes, build communities, and support each other in impactful ways. It's not a one-way street; it's a two-way street where we impact our communities and ensure that no one falls through the cracks. We must connect with those who may not have any other support and authentically take care of them, especially those who are most vulnerable, such as Black, indigenous, and other women of color. While we are facing an overall maternity health crisis, these communities are experiencing it four times worse. By being authentic, advocating for ourselves, and advocating for them, we can lift each other up. If the principles presented can shift the mindset and actions of even one person, the ripple effect will continue, and my purpose here will be fulfilled.

CHAPTER 1

Who Are You?

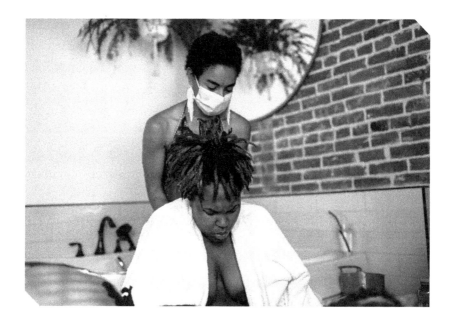

THE IMPORTANCE OF SELF-AWARENESS

When I was a little girl, I carried around my little Cabbage Patch doll, Viola. Everywhere I went, you would find me telling stories to Viola and creating outfits for her. I'd always be carrying my little baby doll. If I wasn't with Viola, you could most certainly find me reading a book or building worm hotels. Layer by layer, I'd dig in the dirt and place worms in a cup. I was a creative child, so it was normal to find me searching my dresser for a pair of jeans to cut up and sew into a dress.

During this season, I must have been nine years old, and my life was consumed with baby dolls, books, and bugs. Looking back, it was a glimpse of what my life would be like one day. As I analyze and reflect upon the trajectory of my life and my roles as a mother, author, birth worker, and placenta specialist, I can say that my inclinations early on now make so much sense.

What does this have to do with identity? When we think about our identity, we tend to think about what people have told us they wanted us to be. However, it is much more than a set of beliefs and mindsets instilled by our families. It's important for us to reflect on our identity, what that means in the scope of our purpose, and what we are meant to do while we are alive and breathing. Now, it is the time to embark on a journey of self-reflection and navigate our inner workings to identify who we are.

First, we must understand several factors that impact our identity. At the core of our identity lies a complex web of variables, including our genetic makeup, cultural background, upbringing, experiences, and relationships. These variables interact with one another in intricate ways, shaping our personality traits, values, beliefs, and attitudes.

Studies in psychology suggest that our identity is formed through a combination of nature and nurture.[1] Genetic makeup plays a significant role in shaping our temperament and innate disposition toward certain behaviors and emotions. For example, some people may be naturally more outgoing and sociable, while others may be more introverted and reflective. However, our genes are not the only determining factor in shaping our identity. Our environment and experiences also play a significant role. From a young age, our upbringing and cultural background shape our worldviews and beliefs, influencing our behavior and choices. For example, someone who grows up in a religious household may have a strong sense of morality and spirituality, while someone from a secular background may prioritize rationality and skepticism.

Furthermore, our relationships and experiences throughout our lives also shape our identity. Our interactions with family, friends, romantic partners, and colleagues all shape our personalities, values, and beliefs. Traumatic experiences can also significantly impact our identity, often leading to significant changes in our behavior and worldview. Understanding these factors can help us better understand ourselves and others.

Sure, experiences, people, and interactions shape who we are. But there are inclinations and innate behaviors that have already been a part of us since birth. They can be seen since childhood, giving us a glimpse of an identity that will unravel, leading us to our purpose and destiny.

Take this moment to reflect on your childhood. How did you express yourself as a little child? What were your interests? What sparked joy in your eyes? If you have the privilege of having loved ones in your life, ask them about who you were as a child. They could help you see yourself through their lens. Listen to how they describe you. What calls your attention most and why?

Having conversations with your grandparents, parents, aunts, or uncles may give you a clear idea about your truest expressions. They can provide authentic insight to help you see a pattern in your life. As we explore our identity and how it manifests itself in birth work, I would like for us to take a minute and reflect on who we were as children and young adolescents.

Audit yourself by asking the following questions:

- What were your interests as a child?

- What were you inclined to do?

- What activities brought the most joy?

- What were you most excited about?

- What did you love to read or watch?

- What made you light up inside?

- What was something you could do for hours and lose track of time?

- What were some challenges and why?

- What were your beliefs about others and the world around you?

These answers could give you clues about how to build a life full of passion, purpose, love, and fulfillment. Each question can help you navigate your deepest thoughts and feelings you never knew were present.

Ask yourself the following five questions and what they represent.

1. What were my favorite activities and hobbies as a child?

   Recalling the activities and hobbies you enjoyed as a child can provide insights into your personality, interests, and talents. Were you drawn to solitary pursuits like reading or drawing, or did you prefer more social activities like team sports or music lessons?

2. Who were my closest friends, and what were they like?

   The friends that we choose as children can provide clues about our social preferences and values. Were you drawn to outgoing and adventurous friends, or did you prefer quieter and more introspective companions?

3. How did I handle challenges and setbacks as a child?

   Examining how you coped with challenges and setbacks as a child can reveal important information about your resilience and coping mechanisms. Did you tend to give up easily or persist in the face of difficulty? Did you seek support from others or try to solve problems independently?

4. What were my earliest memories, and why do I remember them?

   Recalling your earliest memories can be a useful exercise in understanding how your brain processes and retains information.

Examining why you remember certain events can also provide insights into the things that were most important to you as a child.

5. What did I believe about the world, and how has that changed?

Examining your beliefs and attitudes as a child can reveal how your worldview has evolved over time. Did you have a strong sense of justice or empathy for others, or were you more self-centered and focused on your own needs? How have your experiences and interactions with others shaped your current beliefs and values?

As you engage in self-reflection and evaluate your childhood, don't just think about these things. I urge you to write your answers. When you start writing your thoughts, it activates various areas of the brain, including those responsible for language, memory, and emotion. Writing helps to organize and clarify your thoughts, which can have numerous benefits for your mental health and cognitive functioning. Although we're talking about identity within the realm of birth work, I genuinely believe these reflections will help you better understand who you are in relation to every aspect of your life. It will help you go through the layers of your identity, helping you piece together information about yourself that was unknown.

When I think about who I was when I started this journey, I really must laugh. I was a hot-headed, passionate young adult who knew more about what I didn't want and wouldn't allow than about who I was and what I wanted to see in this world. The way I showed up for the families that I supported, including my own, early on was an indication of my nurturing nature.

I kind of smirk to myself because it was very much about protection and ensuring that they were treated with respect and care, and while that hasn't gone away, that intention hasn't changed. That protective and nurturing part of me has always been there from the very beginning. But who I am, how I show up, and how I communicate definitely have—I've experienced growth in beautiful ways. Self-awareness has led me to evolve to be my optimal self.

You must understand that developing self-awareness is a vehicle that will allow you to arrive at a place where you can recognize and understand your own thoughts, feelings, and behaviors. It involves being able to reflect on your experiences, values, and beliefs and how they shape your perceptions of yourself and the world around you.

Self-awareness can lead you to discover your identity by helping you recognize and understand your unique characteristics, strengths, and weaknesses. By reflecting on your past experiences and how they have shaped you, you can identify positive or negative patterns. Self-awareness can also help you identify personal growth and development areas, which is extremely helpful when you are involved in birth work. Because you are a massive source of support during the birthing journey, it's important to be aware of who you are and who others are and learn to identify emotional and physical needs. Believe it or not, self-awareness can help you become intuitive and in tune with others on a deeper level.

When you are a doula and spend your time caring for others, being self-aware can be highly beneficial. Here are some of the benefits:

- *Empathy*: By being aware of your own emotions and experiences, you can better understand the emotions and experiences of others. This can help you to develop empathy and compassion toward the people you are caring for and to provide more personalized and effective support.

- *Boundaries*: Being self-aware can also help you establish healthy boundaries with the people you care for. By understanding your own needs and limitations, you can set appropriate limits on how much emotional and physical energy you give to others.

- *Communication*: Self-awareness can improve your communication skills by helping you understand your communication style and how others perceive it. By being aware of your strengths and weaknesses in communication, you can adapt your approach to better meet the needs of the people you care for.

- *Resilience*: Being self-aware can also improve your resilience in the face of challenging situations. By recognizing your own emotions and stressors, you can take steps to manage them effectively and avoid burnout. This can help you provide consistent and compassionate care to the people you are supporting on their birthing journey.

My ability to be self-aware about how people are experiencing me in various spaces has helped me go a long way in birth work. Walking into various spaces, hospitals, birth centers, and home births over the years, I've become keenly aware of how my energy can influence and/or shift the space that I enter. When we consider that the actual birthing process is one of the most vulnerable experiences that someone will ever live through, it's important to consider our role and be intentional about how we influence that space.

The first step to being self-aware is honesty... Plain old honesty is key, and the ability to be thoughtful beyond yourself and your self-perception. So, as we begin to talk about identity, I'd like for you to filter through, honestly, who you are, why you're doing this work, and how you think you show up. What kind of feedback have people given you over the years about your personality or how they experience you? Then we'll delve into how that can influence your journey as a birth worker.

HOW YOU PRESENT AS A DOULA

When it comes to dealing with Black women and supporting them in the birthing space, number one, it's important to understand how you and your energy are being received. There needs to be a certain level of sensitivity, which I think is useful in all areas of life, but definitely when you are engaging with Black women at birth.

By and large, Black women are hit with statistics left and right about how bringing life into this world can easily become a terrifying and daunting event. What is supposed to be a joyous and celebratory event is often riddled with doubt, fear, and abuse, which snatches the joy out from under us. The statistics, fear, and fearmongering associated with Black women birthing can often be exacerbated by insensitive or ill-equipped birth support.

According to the Centers for Disease Control and Prevention (CDC), Black women are two to three times more likely to experience pregnancy-related complications or death than White women. Black women also have higher rates of preterm birth, low birth weight, and infant mortality compared with other racial and ethnic groups.

Fearmongering related to natural birthing or birthing overall may contribute to these disparities by discouraging women from seeking medical care or making informed choices about their birth experiences. Some examples of fearmongering related to natural birthing may include claims that it is unsafe or increases the risk of complications or death for the mother or baby. This can be particularly harmful to Black women, who may already face higher levels of anxiety and mistrust of medical institutions due to historical and contemporary experiences of racism and discrimination. Instilling fear in Black women can have negative impacts on maternal and infant health outcomes. Thus, being mindful and sensitive to these facts allows you to show up as a source of comfort, care, and a listening ear, and to affirm that you are there to hear the concerns and questions of the family you're supporting.

Doulas play a vital role in providing families with physical, emotional, and informational support during the birthing process. Here are three ways doulas can help support families while also being resourceful:

1. *Providing continuous support*: Doulas can provide continuous support throughout the birthing process, offering physical and emotional support to the laboring person and their partner. This may include techniques such as massage, breathing exercises,

and positions to help manage pain and discomfort. Doulas can also offer emotional support by providing encouragement, reassurance, and a calming presence during what can be a stressful and challenging time.

2. *Offering information and resources*: Doulas can help families make informed decisions by providing them with accurate and up-to-date information about the birthing process, including different options for pain management and interventions. Doulas can also help families access resources such as childbirth education classes, lactation consultants, and other support services to help them prepare for and navigate the postpartum period.

3. *Advocating for families*: Doulas can act as advocates for families, ensuring that their preferences and needs are respected and communicated effectively to medical providers. Doulas can help families understand their rights and options, and work with them to create a birth plan that reflects their preferences and values. Doulas can also help families navigate complex medical systems and procedures, and act as a liaison between families and medical providers to ensure that everyone is on the same page.

Although we are viewed as a source of support and can provide families with the comfort they need throughout the birthing experience, there are factors to consider, such as physical boundaries and family dynamics:

- Doulas and birth workers may encounter situations where they must navigate physical boundaries with their clients. For example, a client may request that the doula provide physical support during birthing, such as holding their hand or rubbing their back. While providing physical support is a crucial part of a doula's role, doulas need to establish clear boundaries and obtain consent from their clients to ensure they are comfortable with the level of physical contact. Also, it is important to read the room when it comes to maintaining physical boundaries with your clients. Every family may not be comfortable sharing their history, whether it involves any physical or sexual trauma, or maybe personal space is just their preference. When engaging with Black women, understand that there are minimal areas of life in which we have autonomy over ourselves and our space. This is an unfortunate part of our life and our experiences overall. But giving birth may be the one opportunity we have to exercise autonomy and care given proper conditions and support.

- Doulas and birth workers may also encounter challenging family dynamics, such as conflicts between partners, disagreements over birth preferences, or cultural or religious differences. Navigating these situations can be uncomfortable and may require the doula to mediate or provide emotional support to all parties involved. As birth workers, we need to establish clear communication with our clients and respect their boundaries and preferences while also providing support and guidance to help navigate challenging moments.

Having a doula present can be the best opportunity to have at least one relationship where our physical, emotional, and spiritual boundaries are respected. But as a birth worker, although you may know that the entire birth experience is beautiful, you must be prepared to navigate uncomfortable situations and learn to adapt to different personalities and characters.

Earlier in my career, I volunteered at a birth where a young lady had struggled with suicidal tendencies. It was a sensitive case that required gentleness, high-level advocacy, and delicate physical boundaries. We hadn't had any prenatal interaction beforehand as it was a last-minute call for support I was volunteering for. When I arrived at the hospital, she was accompanied by her mother and sister. This appeared to be the ideal supportive situation for the average eye. You'd think, "A loving mother and a sister present to support during the birthing process. What more could a girl ask for, right?" But it's a misfire and a long shot. It was an inaccurate depiction of what was taking place.

As she and I communicated quietly by the bed, she informed me that she had a very traumatic and harmful relationship with her mother and sister. According to her, they were overbearing and had made her life "a living hell," as she put it. She stated that they treated her as if she was unable to make any sound decisions on her own and created a hostile environment for her if she made decisions contrary to their desires.

So, what did I do? I scanned her arms and saw the healed scars of times she had harmed herself. I caught the look of desperation in her eyes. She whispered to me that she desired to give birth to her son naturally and wanted to do so with or without her mother and sister in the same room.

In the background, her mother and sister were casually talking about things from food to fashion. They were in their own little world. There came the point where she was being asked about what choices she would like to make regarding an epidural and if she wanted any other interventions. Her mother and sister began to chide her about how weak she was and how she needed to get the medicine because she wouldn't be able to handle the pain.

At that moment, she decided that she wanted to give birth naturally. She looked at me with pleading eyes and said, "PLEASE make them leave." Having assessed their personalities up until that point, I knew that that wasn't something that they would receive well from me as I was the newbie in the room. So, I pulled a nurse aside and let her know what was happening and had her ask them to leave.

As labor progressed, through affirmation and support, I constantly checked in with my client to ask what she needed and asked what touch was okay. During labor, she ended up telling me the story of her life, her relationship with the baby's father, and why he wasn't present. She told me that her dedication to giving birth naturally in that moment was not only about what she wanted for her body but also about a reclamation of autonomy. She was proving a point to her mother and her sister that she was strong enough. It was something she wanted to cherish and also be able to tell her child about how she brought him into the world. This was her moment to be the hero of her own story, and I was grateful to be a part of it.

Understanding your role as a doula is extremely important. You have no idea what giving birth means to your client. You may have no idea what level of empowerment, what new story they're writing for themselves. It's your duty to be tapped in, clear, and give space for whatever that moment requires.

As a doula and birth worker, your role can have a profoundly positive impact on the woman giving birth. Doulas provide emotional, physical, and informational support throughout the birthing process, helping women feel empowered, informed, and supported during one of the most transformative experiences of their lives.

Here are some ways in which doulas can make a difference in the entire birthing experience:

- *Emotional support*: Giving birth can be a highly emotional experience, and having a supportive and compassionate doula can make a significant difference in a woman's emotional well-being. Doulas provide a calming presence, offer encouragement and reassurance, and help women feel more confident in their ability to give birth. By providing a safe and nurturing space, doulas help women feel more comfortable and secure during labor and delivery, which can lead to a more positive birth experience overall.

- *Physical support*: Doulas are trained in various comfort measures and pain-management techniques that can help women manage the physical discomforts of labor and delivery. These may include massage, position changes, breathing exercises, and other techniques that help women feel more comfortable and relaxed during birthing. By helping women manage their pain and discomfort, doulas can help women have a more positive and empowering birth experience.

- *Advocacy and communication*: Doulas can act as advocates for women during labor and delivery, helping them communicate effectively with medical providers and ensuring that their preferences and needs are respected. Doulas can help women understand their options and make informed decisions, and they can also help women navigate complex medical procedures and interventions. By liaising between women and medical providers, doulas can help women feel more informed and in control of their birth experience.

- *Information and education*: Doulas are trained to provide information and education about the birthing process, including different options for pain management and interventions, as well as postpartum care and breastfeeding. By providing women with accurate and up-to-date information, doulas help women make informed decisions and feel more confident in their ability to give birth and care for their newborns.

- *Continuity of care*: Doulas provide continuous support throughout the birthing process, from early labor through delivery and the postpartum period. This continuity of care can help women feel more comfortable and secure, knowing they have a consistent source of support and guidance throughout their birthing experience.

Understanding what stage of life your client is in and paying attention to cues and body language all matter. Even when it comes down to your personal hygiene, making sure that you are showing up in a way that is not overtaking and dominating the space, making sure that you're well-groomed, making sure that your teeth are brushed and that any sort of perfume or scent that you have on isn't overpowering or intense.

Now, in general, this will matter through prenatal, the birth experience, and postpartum care. Number one, because you want to take into consideration the sensitivity of pregnancy hormones. We can smell just the strangest things. The smallest of notes, the pregnancy nose can pick up on. So, when you're entering a space, it's so essential that you start off in a neutral position so that you can learn the family, learn their likes and dislikes, and really get a feel for how you may be able to show up and engage with them.

How is this linked to your identity? As a birth worker, you might receive messaging from places that center you. You are the superhero. You are showing up. You are the central person in this family's story—but I'm here to tell you that's not at all true. You are a huge source of support, so how you show up in your presentation, in your tone of voice, and even in your choice of perfume or not shows whether you can de-center yourself to serve and support others.

Who do you want to be? Do you want to be the person that steps into the room and is unaware that they have filled the entire space with an overpowering scent? Do you want to be the person that does not listen to hear but listens to respond? Do you want to be that person that people just can't wait to open up to because it's like talking to their auntie, sister, or grandmother?

These are all things to consider as you decide who you want to be in this work. You have to audit yourself and identify what you bring to the table and what changes you need to make to be effective and have a positive impact. As a doula, there are several questions you can ask yourself to ensure that you are providing considerate, empathetic, compassionate, and caring support to the families you work with. Here are some examples:

- Am I listening actively to the concerns and needs of the woman and their partner or support team?

- Am I providing information in a clear, understandable way and free from judgment or bias?

- Am I supporting the woman in making informed decisions

about their care and advocating for their wishes and preferences with the care providers?

- Am I showing compassion and empathy for the woman's physical and emotional experiences during labor and birth?

- Am I providing physical comfort measures, such as massage, breathing techniques, or position changes, to help ease the discomfort?

- Am I maintaining a nonjudgmental and non-biased approach to different birth preferences, including medical interventions or non-medical options?

- Am I respecting cultural or religious beliefs and practices and ensuring the family's preferences are integrated into their birth plan?

- Am I supporting the woman and their partner or support team in creating a positive and empowering birth experience, regardless of the outcome?

- Am I respecting the boundaries and limitations of my role as a doula?

- Am I always ensuring that I am providing appropriate and ethical support at all times?

- Am I seeking ongoing education and training to improve my knowledge and skills as a birth worker and stay up-to-date on current evidence-based practices in the field?

By asking yourself these questions, you can ensure that you are providing the highest-quality support to the families you serve. You must be willing to engage in retrospection because it's the only way to improve and evolve into a better individual as a whole. Who you are as a birth worker is important, but who you are as a human being makes all the difference.

Birth work is deeply personal and involves much one-on-one inter-action. When you're thinking about the level of interaction that you're having with a human being that you may have no history with—you may not know them from Adam—it's important to understand that your first impression, second impression, third impression, every single impression matters. It all matters, because every time you have a touch point with your clients, they are thinking, "Oh, this is the person that's going to be there for me when I actually give birth." So, every moment, as much as you're paying attention to their cues and learning about them, they're also deciding whether you are someone they can trust. They are actively thinking and wondering whether or not you are someone they can be vulnerable with, and this is extremely important as you are building your foundation of trust in your relationship with the families you support.

Remember, as a birth worker, the first thing you must work on is establishing a relationship. And as with any relationship, trust is key, especially because the birthing journey is a delicate and sensitive experience. Trust is an essential element in the relationship between a doula and a woman giving birth. Here are some ways in which trust plays an important role:

- *Feeling comfortable and safe*: A woman in labor is often in a vulnerable position and needs to feel comfortable and safe with the people around her. If a woman trusts her doula, she will feel more relaxed and comfortable, which can help facilitate the birthing process.

- *Open communication*: Trust encourages open communication between the doula and the woman giving birth. When there's trust, the woman is more likely to share her fears, concerns, and preferences, which can help the doula provide better support.

- *Support and advocacy*: A doula who has earned the trust of the woman giving birth is more likely to be seen as a supportive and trustworthy ally. This trust can help the doula better advocate for the woman's preferences and needs, leading to a more positive and empowering birth experience.

- *Respect for boundaries*: Trust between a doula and a woman giving birth also involves respect for boundaries. When the doula has earned the woman's trust, she is more likely to respect her wishes and preferences and not overstep her role.

- *Better outcomes*: Studies have shown that when a woman trusts her doula, she is more likely to have a positive birth experience and better outcomes for herself and her baby.[2]

EXAMINING YOUR MOTIVATIONS AND SKILLS

We are all interpersonal beings designed to connect interdependently. And when you are a birth worker and doula, and you connect with families and witness firsthand how life enters this world, it can be the most emotional, spiritual, and fulfilling work you will ever do. So, think about why you do this work. Is it something that you feel that you were called to? If so, were the experiences rooted in trauma? Were they rooted in a beautiful experience that you witnessed or shared? Getting to the root of why you are walking this path is very important to help you shape your identity in birth work.

There are many reasons why women may choose to enter the birthing work and doula field, and there is no particular personality type that is drawn to this work. Here are some of the reasons women may pursue a career as a doula:

- *Passion for childbirth and maternal health*: Many doulas are passionate about childbirth and maternal health and want to support women during this transformative experience.

- *Desire to empower women*: Doulas often see their role as empowering women to make informed decisions about their care and supporting them in achieving their birth preferences.

31

- *Personal experience*: Some women become doulas because they had a positive birth experience themselves and want to help others have the same.

- *Previous career or life experience*: Some women come to doula work after careers in healthcare, social work, or other helping professions, while others may have had life experiences that drew them to supporting women during childbirth.

- *Flexibility*: The doula profession can offer flexibility in terms of work hours and the ability to work independently.

There are many reasons one can pursue this profession, but I will make a note here. If you have personally had a traumatic birth experience, or you have witnessed a traumatic birth experience, and that has given you this fire and passion to become a birth worker, it's a beautiful motivator. If you were encouraged to pursue this field so that no one experiences what you went through, then I encourage you to please take the time to process, discharge, and release the trauma you are dealing with.

You must deal with the trauma you witnessed and/or experienced. Otherwise, you cannot show up fully and support the families waiting for you. Being a birth worker is demanding because you need to be okay in order for you to help others and care for them fully. You must be present and have a healthy state of mind. However, there are reasons or red flags that will help you determine whether or not you are doing your job well. Here are some examples:

- *Lack of experience or training*: Doulas who are inexperienced or have not received adequate training may not have the skills or knowledge needed to support women effectively during childbirth.

- *Personal biases or beliefs*: Doulas who hold personal biases or beliefs that conflict with the preferences of the woman, or their family, may have difficulty providing unbiased support.

- *Overstepping boundaries*: Doulas who overstep their boundaries or try to take control of the birth experience may not be providing the support that the woman and their family need.

- *Poor communication*: Doulas with poor communication skills may struggle to effectively advocate for the woman's needs and preferences or provide the emotional support needed during childbirth.

- *Burnout or stress*: Doulas who experience burnout or high stress levels may not be able to provide the same level of support as they would under normal circumstances.

- *Conflict with care providers*: Doulas who have conflicts with care providers or hospital staff may have difficulty providing effective support to the woman during childbirth.

- *Unforeseen circumstances*: Unforeseen circumstances, such as emergencies or unforeseen medical interventions, may require a doula to adjust their approach or may limit their ability to provide support.

Though we may not want to consider that we may be burned out or have issues with our communication style, or any of the above hindrances, we must be honest with ourselves. You cannot improve or change what you cannot see, which is why I urged you at the beginning of this book to look within and evaluate who you are genuinely. Be open to change and see your weaknesses not as a downfall but as an opportunity for growth. Despite our personal struggles, we must heal, process our issues, and care for our clients from a place without biases and unobstructed views.

As birth workers, one of the most important things to remember is that we are not coming to the table with an agenda of how we want our client's birth to go. We are here to support, show up and help each family achieve their desired birth experience. When pivots are necessary, and sometimes a larger one is required, we are the constant emotional and physical support for them as they navigate the different waves and changes they will experience at birth.

When the birth experience does not go as planned or expected, birth workers can help tremendously by providing emotional and practical support to women and their families. You can provide emotional support by listening to the woman's concerns and fears, offering reassurance and encouragement, and helping her process her feelings about the experience. You can also provide practical support, such as helping the woman find a comfortable position, providing water or snacks, or assisting with relaxation techniques. With your knowledge, you can give the right information and support to help the woman and her partner make informed decisions about their care, including weighing the risks and benefits of different options. You can even assist with breastfeeding support and guide postpartum care and recovery. The goal is to help women and their families in every way you can, which is why you need to become self-aware, mindful, and knowledgeable.

Birth work is meaningful and purposeful. Think about why you do what you do. What is grounding you in your birth work practice? Is this something you're doing because it's a fad, and you saw many videos on YouTube, or would you really consider building a life on it? Is this important? Yes.

Develop clarity as to why you do what you do. Because your "why" can lead you to live a fulfilled life or can lead to burnout and exhaustion. You won't be happy, which can negatively affect those you serve and care for. If you are saying one thing out of your mouth about why you're doing this work and it's not actually congruent with the real reason that you're doing this work, it will show up as inauthentic in spaces where you're trying to secure clients or create content around birth work.

It's very important that your true desires are congruent with how you're actually showing up. What do I mean? If you are a mother who wants to share her experience about your birth and you decide, "Hey, I want to become a doula. I want to talk more about the impact of birth work," but you don't really think that you'll be able to be a hands-on practitioner of this work, there are other ways to become an advocate or creatively share your passions and stories of impact.

Some areas of birth work are more content-heavy, but if you actually go, and you just jump in, and you say, "Oh, I should attend a birth because this is something I'm really passionate about," if that's not actually congruent and doesn't match your true heart's desire of how you need to and/or want to show up in this work, that will show in the dynamic between you and the family that you're seeking to serve—this is a recipe for disaster.

Broken people break people. Without processing any sort of trauma or unresolved anger or disappointment with your own childbirth experience, or the birth that you have witnessed, you leave space to show up in a way that could potentially be traumatic for the families you seek to serve. Your reactions could be more intense than they need to be. They could be more passive than they need to be. You can hyper-focus on certain subjects and things simply based on the trauma you experienced versus approaching your support based upon the actual situation in front of you, the actual family in front of you, their list of concerns, and their particular background.

Personal trauma can have a significant impact on the work a doula does. Trauma can be defined as an experience that overwhelms an individual's ability to cope, leaving them feeling helpless, out of control, and vulnerable. If a doula has experienced trauma in their own life, it can affect how they approach their work with women and families during childbirth. The following are some ways personal trauma can affect the work you do as a doula:

- *Triggers and emotional reactions*: Trauma can cause triggers or emotional reactions that make it difficult for a doula to provide adequate support. For example, if you have experienced a traumatic birth, you may find it challenging to remain present and calm during a difficult birth.

- *Difficulty connecting with clients*: Trauma can also affect your ability to connect with clients and build rapport. If you are struggling with your own trauma, you may have difficulty being fully present and empathetic with your clients.

- *Personal biases and beliefs*: Trauma can also influence a doula's biases and beliefs about childbirth, which can affect their care. For example, a doula who has experienced trauma during childbirth may hold beliefs that lead them to advocate for certain types of interventions or to avoid certain birthing scenarios.

- *Burnout and self-care*: Trauma can also contribute to burnout and exhaustion, making it difficult for a doula to continue providing effective support over time. Doulas who have experienced trauma may need to take extra steps to prioritize their self-care and well-being to continue working effectively with women and families.

If you can identify yourself and detect that you feel any of the above, it's important to take steps to address the impact it may have on your work, such as seeking support from a therapist or supervisor, practicing self-care, and being transparent with clients about your experiences and how they may affect the work you do. By doing so, you can continue to provide compassionate and positive support to women and families during childbirth.

In almost every area of life, Black women have been conditioned to be silent. Many people have this misconception that women will stand up and speak when they feel a certain way. But that is not always the case. You might think that if a woman feels uncomfortable, then they'll just say something, but it's not true. I'm telling you now that, as Black women, we are conditioned not to speak up. We are taught not to rock the boat and are discouraged from expressing discomfort about something. We are raised and conditioned to believe and respond in this way to preserve other folks' feelings.

In other words, we must be mindful of what others feel at the cost of suppressing our own feelings and thoughts. We are used to institutions, systems, and people exerting themselves as the authority over our emotions, feelings, and even the sensations in our bodies. In the medical industrial complex, we're used to being dismissed when we're reporting pain or discomfort. We are used to being silenced and being treated as the person that is not the expert on our body when we're in certain spaces, and this can trickle from our family dynamics to our relationship dynamics to the dynamics with different professionals, doctors, midwives, and OB-GYNs in our life.

As a birth worker, what you do is not just another role. The Black women and families you support and help, need to be empowered to break the silence and speak for themselves. Start seeing the grand picture. Your role as a birth worker is a lifetime opportunity to be, perhaps, the one person in another woman's life who will listen, who will empower, who will affirm, who will encourage them to speak up for themselves, to get in tune with their bodies, and to be clear in their communication about what feels good, what doesn't, what's working, and what's not. You can ensure that you advocate for them to learn how to self-advocate for themselves. Again, doulas are not saviors but serve and become a great source of comfort and peace amid the painful and uncertain waves of pregnancy and giving birth.

Our job is to empower, affirm, and support families all along their birthing journey. If your identity is rooted in being right, being the expert, and forcing people to do things they don't want to do, this may not be the path for you.

Here are four skills and habits that can help you become the best you can be:

1. *Active listening*: Active listening is crucial because it allows you to truly understand your client's needs, concerns, and desires. When you actively listen to your clients, you can provide more personalized and practical support.

2. *Empathy*: Empathy is the ability to understand and share the feelings of others. By being empathetic, you can validate your client's emotions and experiences, helping them feel heard and supported. Emotional validation is important.

3. *Flexibility and adaptability*: Childbirth can be unpredictable, and the more flexible and adaptable you are, the more you can provide the best possible support. You can make a difference by adjusting to changing circumstances and individual client needs.

4. *Continuous learning and professional development*: The best doulas are those who are committed to continuous learning and professional development. This includes staying up-to-date on the latest research, attending workshops, and training programs, and seeking feedback from clients and peers to improve their skills and knowledge continually.

Above all, the foundation to being the best birth worker you can be is honesty, thoughtfulness, and self-reflection as we embark on this journey of being the support families need during childbirth.

NOTES

1   For example: Honeycutt, H. (2019, September 30) "Nature and nurture as an enduring tension in the history of psychology." *Oxford Research Encyclopedia of Psychology.* https://oxfordre.com/psychology/view/10.1093/acrefore/9780190236557.001.0001/acrefore-9780190236557-e-518.

2   For example: O'Rourke, K., Yelland, J., Newton, M., and Shafiei, T. (2022) "How and when doula support increases confidence in women experiencing socioeconomic adversity: Findings from a realist evaluation of an Australian volunteer doula program." *PloS One 17*, 6, e0270755. doi:10.1371/journal.pone.0270755

CHAPTER 2

The Impact of Self-Development

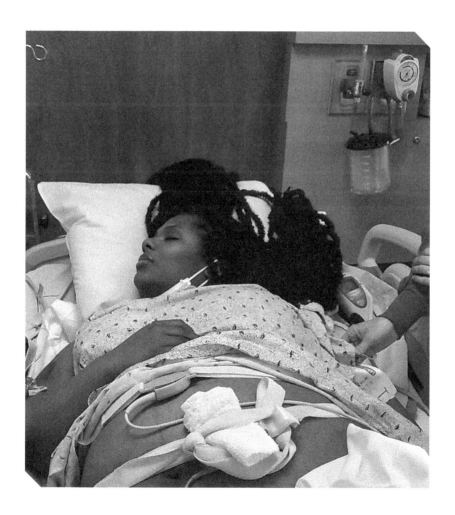

I remember the phone call like it was yesterday. A client and her husband reached out to me to support them during the pregnancy of their rainbow baby. It was a sensitive time for them, and while interviewing me they needed to know that I would hold space for them on this journey, that we were a good spiritual match, and that I would honor the space of each family member important to them. One of the things that struck me was the mother's personal journey of growth and understanding. She had been the first to do things differently in her family in many areas, so too with her birth choices. She was the first person in several generations to birth naturally and vaginally. In her country, it is customary to schedule c-sections automatically regardless of medical necessity. Being the firecracker she is, she decided to do things her own way. She and her husband settled on birthing naturally in a birth center.

One of the most impactful moments I remember was right before their baby entered the world. Her mother had flown in from South Africa, her husband was by her side supporting her every step of the way, and as her doula I was reading verses of encouragement by her side as she gave birth. I glanced around the room, and I saw her mother slowly pacing back and forth at her bedside. I knew that she was nervous and unfamiliar with the birthing process she was witnessing. As my client pushed, and birthed her child I witnessed the awe and joy on her mother's face. Her personal journey, personal development, and healing all culminated in that moment. For this family, there were new options, new ways of doing things, because of her bravery. Be Brave.

Anyone that knows me knows that I am dedicated to radical growth. Over the years, my healing journey, birth work journey, and parenting journey have been intertwined. In recent years, my ability to have mental toughness has expanded. My capacity to communicate and stay focused during hard times has increased, but this hasn't come without much work. Self-development and improvement aren't accidental. It takes a continuous flow of small decisions that compound into massive results over time.

MINDSET AND MENTAL TOUGHNESS

Your mindset is everything because it consists of your beliefs. And everything you do derives from who you believe you are. When you wrestle with limiting beliefs, things get complicated. Your own thoughts and lack of belief in yourself will lead you to make agreements that do not serve you long-term. Examples of some of the negative agreements that we make are:

- We cling to believing that we are not good enough.

- We choose to delay our progress due to lack of discipline.

- We don't view ourselves as worthy.

- We believe we are useless and incompetent.

- We don't think we have what it takes.

- We think we're helpless.

When we agree to believe such perspectives about ourselves, we are setting ourselves up for all kinds of failures and setbacks. Life is hard enough as it is. We must create a healthy mindset and cultivate healthy thoughts. Although negative thoughts will always emerge, and we will battle with self-doubt, the best way to overcome these hurdles is to overpower them with actions. You cannot wait to be confident; you have to move and make bold decisions despite the doubts you fear. As you do so, you will gain confidence in what you do, especially in the field of birth work.

Your mindset is everything and if you are to cultivate inner strength you have to seek it and put in the work. If so, this is your chance to reset and make things new. Developing a strong mindset and mental toughness is essential for achieving your goals and reaching success in your career and calling. It takes time, effort, and consistency to acquire these skills, but the results will be well worth it.

The first thing you can do is define your goals. The best way to define your goals is to be clear and specific about what you want to achieve. This will help you focus your energy and efforts on what matters most to you. Start by breaking down your bigger goals into smaller, achievable objectives. Set short-term goals that are realistic and can be accomplished in a reasonable amount of time. These smaller goals should lead you to the larger ones. Long-term goals are just as important. Make sure they are challenging, but still achievable. Think long-term to identify strategies and solutions that you can use over the course of your journey to success.

A strong mindset starts with being clear about what it is you want to achieve and understanding how to get there. Once you have determined your goals, you can create a plan for reaching them and move forward with confidence and determination. As I mentioned previously, if you want to see massive changes in your life you must change your self-talk and changing your self-talk is one of the most important steps to developing a strong mindset and mental toughness. Self-talk is the inner dialogue we have with ourselves, and it's one of the most powerful forces in our lives—it dictates what we do and the outcomes we get. Negative self-talk can be very detrimental to our success and well-being, while positive self-talk can help foster a strong mindset and mental toughness.

To transform your self-talk and develop a strong mindset and mental toughness, here are three key ways to foster positive self-talk:

1. *Identify your negative thoughts*: The first step is to identify any negative thoughts you may have. This can be done by monitoring your internal dialogue and being mindful of how you talk to yourself. Once you've identified these negative thoughts, you can start replacing them with more positive ones. How you talk to yourself can impact how you treat others. Our inner speech emanates vibes and energy. Therefore, we must watch that energy and learn to balance it.

2. *Reframe negative thoughts*: The next step is to reframe any negative thoughts into positive ones. For example, if you have a

negative thought such as "I'm not good enough," reframe it into "I am capable of doing anything I put my mind to." Doing this will help reprogram your brain to think positively. You have to develop new ways for your brain to cope and respond to negative ideas, perspectives, and inner beliefs.

3. *Practice positive affirmations*: Lastly, practice positive affirmations on a daily basis. Positive affirmations are positive statements that help reprogram your mind and focus on what you want in life. Examples of positive affirmations include "I am strong and capable" or "I am confident in my abilities." Writing down your positive affirmations and reading them out loud is a great way to keep them top of your mind throughout the day.

Although it will take time and practice with consistent effort, you can start transforming your self-talk and unlock your potential, especially in birth work and with the clients in your care.

One thing that people don't talk about enough is the power of visualization and how it strengthens your mind. Visualization is a powerful tool that can be used to increase focus and motivation while working toward a goal. It involves creating mental images of the desired outcome, allowing you to picture success. When you practice visualization, you are training your brain to think in a more positive and productive way.

By visualizing yourself succeeding and overcoming obstacles, you are effectively strengthening your willpower and resilience. You can also use visualization as a way to calm yourself down during moments of stress or anxiety while you are in the middle of helping families and are dealing with stressful situations. The goal is to create a clear image in your mind of what you want to accomplish and to stay focused on that image.

To practice visualization, start by finding a quiet place where you can sit comfortably and close your eyes. Take some deep breaths and imagine yourself in a place that brings you peace and relaxation. Then, begin to visualize the outcome of your goals and aspirations. Picture yourself succeeding in whatever it is that you're striving for—being successful in your career, achieving a personal record in sports, or learning something new. Focus on the details of the scene: the colors, the sounds, the smells. Imagine how it will feel when you reach your goals.

When practicing visualization, it's important to remain positive and avoid negative thoughts. Focus on positive outcomes, no matter how small they may seem. Visualization helps to strengthen our self-discipline and increase our confidence, which are essential components of having a strong mindset and developing mental toughness.

Another aspect that we must consider when we think about mental toughness is the need to be resilient in the face of setbacks. Resilience is essential to having a strong mindset and becoming mentally tough. The truth is that you will face many speed bumps along your journey as a doula. You will encounter difficult interactions and moments, making it even more imperative to be resilient no matter what comes your way.

Resilience is the ability to withstand and recover quickly from difficult or challenging situations, the ability to bounce back. When life throws you a curveball, resilience allows you to adapt and move forward in a positive way. How you adapt to what happens will determine the outcome of your experience with families and their birthing experience too. Developing resilience involves building mental and emotional strength so that you can take on the challenge with determination and come out stronger on the other side. Here are some tips to help you become more resilient when faced with setbacks:

- *Acknowledge your emotions*: It's okay to feel overwhelmed, scared, or angry when faced with a setback. Acknowledge these feelings and allow yourself time to process them.

- *Don't give up*: When faced with a setback, it's easy to feel like throwing in the towel. But instead of giving up, focus on what you can do to move forward and find solutions.

- *Re-frame*: Find the opportunity in the situation and look for ways to turn it around. Focusing on the positives and the potential for growth can help you find motivation to move on.

- *Practice self-care*: Take care of yourself during difficult times by eating well, getting enough sleep, exercising, and taking breaks. This will help to keep your mental and emotional health in check, enabling you to better cope with the situation. So, do something for yourself every day, as little as it may be.

- *Get support*: Sometimes, we just need to talk things out or seek advice from someone we trust. Talking to friends and family or seeking professional help if needed can be immensely helpful in providing clarity, perspective, and the motivation to take action. Remember, you are not meant to do life alone. Build a strong support system outside of birth work and in the field. It will help you live a more fulfilled life and will provide the encouragement you need in your moments of weakness.

- *Take action*: Taking action is key to moving forward and finding solutions. Even if you don't have all the answers yet, taking small steps toward a resolution can be incredibly empowering and will help you get closer to overcoming the setback.

By developing your resilience, you can learn how to better handle any unexpected obstacles that come your way and become mentally tough. Keep in mind that setbacks are part of life, but they don't have to define you. Instead, use them as opportunities for growth and development. Embrace obstacles as challenges.

One way to embrace the obstacles you face in the birth work field is to reframe your mindset. Instead of seeing challenges as insurmountable barriers, view them as opportunities for growth and development. Remind yourself that these challenges are helping to strengthen your resolve and make you more capable of handling future challenges with greater success.

When you start to feel overwhelmed, breaking down the challenge into smaller tasks can be helpful. This will help to make the task seem less daunting and more manageable. Acknowledge that there may be times when the challenge will become too much and that it's okay to take a step back and reassess the situation.

It is also important to surround yourself with a supportive team of professionals or friends who can provide encouragement and guidance during difficult times. Having people to lean on and get advice from will help to lighten the load and provide a sense of camaraderie in the face of adversity.

Finally, remember to celebrate your successes as you help women and their families. No matter how small they may seem, be proud of yourself. This will help keep you motivated and resilient as you navigate the many obstacles that come along with birth work.

And I know more than anyone that it's hard to be strong when dealing with your own turmoil and problems, and it may be hard to stay positive. But if you want to develop mental toughness, you must seek ways to stay positive no matter what's happening all around you. This can be easier said than done, especially when life throws us curveballs and we face unexpected obstacles. Here are three ways to stay positive daily:

- *Practice gratitude*: Taking time out each day to reflect on what we are thankful for can help us keep our minds in a positive frame. Write it down, journal it, or put it on your wall or on sticky notes. Do whatever it takes to remind yourself of the good things in your life. Not only will this practice give you a sense of perspective, but it will also remind you of the many blessings we have in our lives.

- *Surround yourself with positive people*: Being around people who support our goals, lift us up, and encourage us can greatly impact our mindset. When we're struggling to stay positive, having someone who will remind us of our strength and potential can be invaluable.

- *Focus on solutions*: Problems are a part of life, but how we approach them can make all the difference. Instead of getting caught up in the drama and the details of a problem, try to focus on the solutions. Thinking about solutions helps us stay positive and take action toward a better future.

These are just a few good practices that can help us stay positive. It's important to remember that staying positive isn't always easy, but with practice, it can become easier. A strong mindset starts with a positive attitude, so make sure you take care of yourself and focus on solutions instead of dwelling on problems.

You have a decision to make whether you like it or not. You must choose to persevere or stay stuck in a place of discontent and discomfort. I hope that you choose perseverance, even if it will demand everything from you. One way to persevere amid a tough time is to focus on what you can control. Instead of being overwhelmed by the negativity and frustration around you, focus on the aspects of your life that you can control. This could be something as simple as choosing to react to a situation positively or opening yourself up to seeing things from a different perspective.

For example, if you're dealing with a difficult client, instead of getting angry or frustrated, consider what you can do to make the situation better. Could you be more organized? Could you be more helpful? Are there any small changes you could make to improve the situation? By focusing on what you can control and being pro-active in changing it, you will build resilience and be more likely to persevere.

Another way to persevere is to take regular breaks. When we're in the midst of a tough time, it can be easy to burn out quickly. Taking regular breaks helps us recharge and gives us the energy to keep going. Whether it's taking a few minutes each day to relax or scheduling a weekend away from work, taking breaks will help keep you mentally strong and able to persevere through even the toughest times. Though you may find it difficult to take breaks, they are vital to your overall well-being because you need to rest and recharge yourself. You must take care of yourself and be okay before you can take care of others.

It's important to remember that no matter how tough things get, there will always be light at the end of the tunnel. Focus on that light and use it as motivation to keep going. Believe in yourself and your ability to make it through this tough period and find success in the future. No matter how tough it gets, don't forget that you have the strength and resilience to persevere.

The most important step in developing a strong mindset is taking action. Taking action is the key to achieving any goal. When faced with an obstacle, don't freeze and let fear take over; instead, take action and move forward. Make a plan, set goals, and develop a strategy. Break down your goals into small achievable tasks and focus on making progress. Be persistent and never give up. Don't be afraid to ask for help when needed, and don't let other people's opinions or negative thoughts distract you from your goal. Focus on the end result and take action to get there. Taking action can be intimidating, but the rewards are worth it. Keep pushing and remind yourself that success is worth the effort.

It's easy to say that the core of mental toughness is the ability to never give up, but it's hard to actually put it into practice. However, if you are willing to commit yourself and stay focused on your goals, no matter how difficult things get, then you will have what it takes to become mentally tough.

When life throws a challenge your way, remind yourself why you are pursuing your career and remember that it's going to take hard work and dedication. Don't give in to negativity or doubt; instead, take each setback as an opportunity to learn and grow. One of the most essential tools in your arsenal is self-discipline. Being able to discipline yourself to stick with a task until you see it through to the end is a key factor in becoming mentally tough. If you find yourself slipping into a negative mindset, use self-talk to snap yourself out of it and refocus on your goals.

Always remind yourself that anything worth achieving will take time and effort, so don't expect immediate success or results. Take it one step at a time and one family at a time. Don't let failure define you. Instead, use failure as a learning experience and keep pushing forward. Remember, the only way you can fail is if you give up. So don't give up, and never stop believing in yourself!

In my mindset practice, one of the foundational pieces of mental toughness has been getting comfortable with being uncomfortable. Not only is this something that I teach my clients to help them navigate the difficulties and discomforts of pregnancy, but it's something I personally do. As a birth worker, I have had to use it so that I could navigate the different ups and downs that I might be met with while I'm supporting a family in birth.

One of the most uncomfortable things you will experience in the field is having to have difficult conversations where you know apprehension can arise, or when you know someone will get defensive. Or maybe you know the reaction of disappointment that's coming. From the get-go, I have to let you know that you need to be okay with discomfort.

The way that I see it and from my experience, when I can create the capacity to have difficult conversations, there's space for me to get things done and help those I'm called to support and help. Accepting uncomfortable situations helps me interact with medical staff or family members who might be presenting in a challenging way while supporting my families. This also allows me to deal with difficult or emotional conversations I need to have with my clients to help them process whatever they're experiencing at any moment.

Without growing my capacity with mental toughness, I would be washed to and from while supporting each family; because each family has a different background, a different challenge, different birth experience, you never know what you're going to get, literally, like a box of chocolates. So, it's important that your mindset and capacity to process and have hard conversations is shored up.

Mental toughness is a concept that I have recently been introduced to, and I can't say that it's something that I can recall utilizing outside of sports. However, I will say that ever since I've been intentional about processing life's experiences that appear to be very difficult, through this lens of mental toughness, it has made life much more peaceful and has given me more clarity and clear perspectives. So, when you have clarity of perspective, it helps to clear the lens of your judgment and even the advice you're giving.

You're not listening through past experiences, unless you're looking for similarities and where you can give recommendations. You're not listening through the traumas and the pain that you've experienced in the past. You have to put everything aside because you are listening to hear the person in front of you, and to advocate and support them in helpful ways, particularly for them.

Overall, mental toughness is a positive trait that can help individuals overcome adversity and achieve their goals. Mental toughness is generally seen as a combination of resilience, grit, determination, and the ability to stay focused under pressure. However, some view it as a negative trait, associating it with an emphasis on competition and winning at all costs. They may see mental toughness as an unrealistic and harmful expectation that can lead to burnout, stress, and mental health problems. But from my experience, mental toughness has made me more resilient and less likely to respond inadequately, say, or do the wrong thing. So, keep doing the things that I expressed before— setting goals, practicing resilience, and cultivating a positive attitude. However, there are three more things you can also add to that list.

- *Develop self-discipline*: Mental toughness requires self-discipline and staying focused on long-term goals. Develop self-discipline by setting a routine, prioritizing time, and avoiding distractions. Yes, you've heard it before, but I want you to look at self-discipline as your ability to establish self-governance. You have what it takes to govern yourself to the point where you are disciplined in every area of life. You are that powerful and have access to have full dominion over your actions and thoughts.

- *Manage stress*: Mental toughness requires the ability to manage stress effectively. Practice stress-management techniques such as deep breathing, meditation, and physical exercise.

- *Seek support*: Being mentally tough doesn't mean not asking or seeking help when you need it. In fact, mental toughness doesn't mean doing things on your own, completely isolated from others. Seek support from a mental health professional when needed. Many people hear the words mental health professional, and they automatically think "crazy." But that's far from being true. Mental health professionals are there to help you process your emotions, put a name to what you are going through, and help equip you with the right coping strategies so that you can have peace and joy in the middle of any situation.

Though it's easier said than done, these strategies can help you when you incorporate them into your daily life. The more you develop yourself, the better the person you become. The better you become, the better you can support others. Thus, it's imperative for you to work on yourself.

Now, I know we've all heard about the importance of serving from a full cup, but we can also take that same thought and apply it to our minds. But how can we fill our minds if we do not understand what we need?

We must work on navigating our thought lives and understanding our thought patterns, managing stress, our moods, and our ability to be disciplined. Our mindset is something that needs continuous work and improvement. In order for us to be a strong and solid support, we have to have a strong and solid mental capacity, to give our mind the proper maintenance and renewal so that we can start pouring out and supporting others. Now, you may be presented with lots of information about each family you support. Add to that the fact that you are dealing with your own personal life and challenges.

You're dealing with internal battles, conflicts, and situational issues that can impact your mood and, in turn, will impact your clients. There are many variables to consider, and the best way to get a handle on the fluctuations of thoughts and emotions is to gain mental clarity. One of the best ways to achieve this is through the art of journaling. Writing daily before you start your day can help you dump all your worries and anxiety-filled thoughts. This process will help you release emotions and tension, and you can welcome positive affirmations and begin incorporating positive self-talk. That way, you will be well on your way to improving your mood, and it's from a place of peace and strength that you can serve those who need your support, such as your clients and colleagues. You must serve from a balanced mindset.

As I know you know, doulas are the physical and emotional constant support for a family. So, whether or not their doctor or midwife is balanced, whether or not their partner or husband is balanced, whether or not their children or mother and mother-in-law are balanced, you, my friend, are in position to be balanced. You are responsible for being strong, solid, consistent support, and it starts with taking care of you.

Frontline workers are people that work directly with the public. We are directly interacting with the public on a consistent basis. If you are supporting a family in a hospital birth, you are just as close, if not closer, to the family as the nurse that is coming and checking vitals, as the midwife or OB that is coming in to help support the birth of the baby. With that being said, making sure that you and your body are strong is an understatement. It's important to be mindful about how stressors affect your hormones and your body as you are supporting others.

Many frontline workers typically neglect their own physical care and pour their energy and effort into their caregiving and service-based support. This is not healthy, and ultimately, it will lead to imbalance. Strengthening your body and being mindful of stress in your body is something that is extremely key. Physical activity, focusing on healthy nutrition, and being clear on your own levels, is something that's going to be of the utmost importance. Understanding your physical baseline is something that will help you to meter out what you actually have a physical capacity to do in birth.

Having had many experiences of birth, I'm here to tell you that some are more physically demanding than others. For instance, if you find that the demographic of families you want to support will be primarily hospital clients, who prefer an epidural, you may find that your birth support is less physically vigorous than the doula that decides that they are going to strictly support natural home-birth families. Just the same, if you decide to support families in a birthing center who also are planning unmedicated birth, your physical activity may or may not be at a high level, but it's important to understand that you will be engaging more heavily with families.

When we think about the hip squeezes, and we think about the rebozo and counter-pressure, we have to account for that impact on our own physical bodies. Now, I'm not saying that you need to be in tip-top shape to be a birth worker or to support a family, but it is extremely important to be mindful of your baseline and what capacity you have physically to support the family. Making sure that you stretch, making sure that your nutrition is depositing vitamins and minerals into your body that you need, that will sustain you should you be attending a 30-hour birth, these are all things that are consistent. Again, over time, your body will wear down, and without a level of intentionality and practice behind treating your body well and strengthening your body in preparation for birth support, you might very well be doing yourself a disservice down the line.

SPIRITUAL GROUNDING

Upon feeling worn out and experiencing burnout, what can you do? You can acknowledge your spirit and soul and know that you have to nurture and take care of it. There is a physical aspect to our lives, but also a spiritual side. Consistently strengthening your spiritual life will allow you proper perspective, language, and the ability to activate areas of your brain that are needed to connect deeply with your clients. We'll spend some time here laying the foundation of spiritual grounding, but we will explore a bit deeper in Chapter 7.

When you are a grounded individual, no matter your spiritual practice, there's a level of calm and peace that you're able to bring to spaces on a consistent basis. Grounding oneself is an important spiritual practice that can be beneficial to one's mental, emotional, and physical health. It is a technique used to help individuals become more connected to themselves, their environment, and the energy that exists within it. Grounding provides an opportunity for people to become more aware of their body and how it interacts with the world around them. It is an essential component in your life.

Defining spiritual grounding is easy. It is a practice that helps to connect and reconnect individuals with the natural energy of the Earth. It is not a religious practice, but rather it encourages an individual to become aware of their connection to the divine and the world around them. Through spiritual grounding, one can feel centered, balanced, and connected to the larger environment.

Spiritual grounding is important for overall well-being because it allows us to release stress, tension, and negative energy that we accumulate in our daily lives. It also helps us to become more mindful and present in our lives, allowing us to be fully present for all of life's moments, both good and bad. Additionally, it can help us to make better decisions and stay in alignment with our highest purpose. It helps to keep us from becoming stuck in our heads or lost in our emotions. Lastly, spiritual grounding can help to cultivate spiritual growth, allowing us to tap into the deep wisdom within ourselves and our environment. And at the end of the day, we need all the wisdom we can have because the situations we will find ourselves in will benefit from it.

Why is spiritual grounding important? Spiritual grounding is an important concept for doulas and birth workers to understand, as it can have a powerful impact on how they practice and how they are able to support their clients. Being spiritually grounded is about finding the connection between your inner self and the universal energies around you, so that you can be more centered in your being.

The level of importance for spiritual grounding cannot be

overstated for those who work with birthing people, as it helps to create a calm and safe environment for both the doula and the birthing person. Grounding yourself spiritually helps to open up the pathways of communication between the two of you, allowing you to work together more effectively.

The spiritual grounding of the birth worker can also have a positive impact on the birthing experience of their client. A spiritually grounded doula has the ability to recognize and access the energy of their client's body, helping to provide a space where the birthing person feels supported and empowered. The doula's own spiritual grounding can also help to create a sense of balance and harmony for the birthing person, which can result in a more positive birth experience.

Ultimately, spiritual grounding is an important practice for doulas and birth workers to understand in order to provide the best possible care to their clients. By being grounded spiritually, doulas can create an environment of safety and trust, while also helping to empower their birthing people.

But you may be wondering how you can ground yourself spiritually. Spiritual grounding is an important aspect of personal growth, as it helps to bring balance, harmony, and joy into our lives. And I always advise you to keep moving forward toward growth. Spiritual grounding helps us to stay connected to our higher self and the universe, which allows us to live in alignment with our true purpose and our highest potential.

When it comes to becoming spiritually grounded, there is a variety of disciplines and strategies that can help us reach this state. For example, meditation, yoga, breathing exercises, and even journaling can all help us achieve spiritual grounding. It's important to find the techniques that work best for you as an individual, as what works for one person may not necessarily work for another.

In addition to using certain techniques to ground yourself spiritually, it's also important to set aside time each day for spiritual practice. This could involve simply taking a few moments for reflection or dedicating an entire hour to meditating or engaging in other spiritual activities. Another beneficial activity is to practice self-care regularly in order to keep our energy levels up and maintain a healthy mindset.

Studies have found that spiritual grounding has numerous benefits for those who practice it.[1] People who engage in regular spiritual practices tend to experience a greater sense of connection and purpose in their lives, as well as improved physical health and emotional well-being. Spiritual grounding can also help improve our ability to focus and concentrate, while also improving relationships with others.

Overall, spiritual grounding is an important part of self-care that can help us remain connected to our true selves and live in alignment with our higher purpose. It can help you become the most authentic version of yourself. By making use of certain disciplines and techniques, as well as setting aside time each day for spiritual practice, we can reap the many benefits of spiritual grounding.

Let's be real. Everyone has challenges in their personal life, and everyone is at different places on their spiritual walk. However, intentionally having a grounded practice that you are continuously developing and growing in is something that will not only benefit you and your family, but it will also benefit everyone involved in the birthing process, including physicians, doctors, and nurses.

Studies have shown that when people have a solid spiritual practice, the parts of our personality and brains that cause us to be more judgmental, and to be sharper and quicker to react, are diminished.[2] That's connected to that area I mentioned about being calmer and being more peaceful. Meditation and prayer have been known to reverse the effects of even cancer.[3] Talking about the impact of your being in a calm and peaceful state while you serve and support others, further expands your ability to be a consistent physical and emotional support.

Without mental, physical, and spiritual self-development, your capacity and growth will ultimately be stunted. As human beings, we are ever-evolving. Every area of our life that we choose to invest in, and to develop and grow, shows a benefit in a totally unrelated area of life. As you develop as an individual, as you grow, as you nourish yourself, mind, body, and soul, you will see the positive benefit show up in who you are as a birth worker and who you are as a person.

NOTES

1   For example: Manning, L., Ferris, M., Rosario, C. N., Prues, M., and Bouchard, L. (2019) "Spiritual resilience: Understanding the protection and promotion of well-being in the later life." *Journal of Religion, Spirituality & Aging* 31, 2, 168–186.

2   Penman J. (2021) "Cognitive and behavioral changes arising from spirituality." *Journal of Religion and Health* 60, 6, 4082–4096. Ryff C.D. (2021) "Spirituality and well-being: Theory, science, and the nature connection." *Religions* 12, 11, 914.

3   For example: Kalir, T. (2023). "The Effect of Mindfulness Techniques on Immune Function in Cancer Patients." In: Rezaei, N. (eds) *Handbook of Cancer and Immunology.* Springer, Cham. https://doi.org/10.1007/978-3-030-80962-1_353-1

     Johns, S. A., Beck-Coon, K., Stutz, P. V., Talib, T. L. *et al.* (2020) "Mindfulness Training Supports Quality of Life and Advance Care Planning in Adults With Metastatic Cancer and Their Caregivers: Results of a Pilot Study." *Am J Hosp Palliat Care,* 37, 2, 88–99.

     Poletti, S., Razzini, G., Ferrari, R., Ricchieri, M. P. *et al.* (2019) "Mindfulness-Based stress reduction in early palliative care for people with metastatic cancer: A mixed-method study." *Complementary Therapies in Medicine,* 47. https://doi.org/10.1016/j.ctim.2019.102218

CHAPTER 3

Beyond Credentials

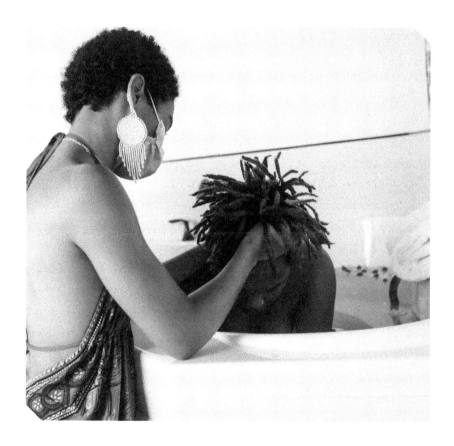

The history of midwifery in America is tricky. Like so many other areas it's nuanced. As a Black and indigenous woman who descended from grand midwives, doctors, farmers, and healers, I understand the difficulty in seeking validation for what already belongs to me. My entry into this work was nontraditional. As a young girl fresh out of high school, one of the most important things to me was my friends. Growing up, my friends were like family, siblings even. When my childhood friend became pregnant a year after we graduated high school, we were all excited and a little afraid.

During her pregnancy there were lots of times where I saw my friend being pushed into the background while her belly, her baby, somehow became the focus. In hindsight, I can say that watching this happen had less to do with some deep, meaningful honor for pregnancy and more to do with wanting my friend to feel loved. Throughout her pregnancy we would hang out just as we would before she was pregnant. When it came time to deliver, her entire family, her child's father, and myself were all at the hospital. I won't get into the details of that experience because it is not my story to tell. Just know that holding space for my friend in intimate moments after her birth and throughout her pregnancy were what initiated me into birth work.

On that day, a birth worker was born. I had no idea what a doula was, I just knew I wanted my friends and family to be supported, advocated for, and doted on during their pregnancy and birth experiences. It would be over ten years later that I'd attend a doula training and become a certified birth doula. At the time of this writing, I have been attending births for over 20 years; for only half of that time have I been trained, certified, and credentialed. There are many insights and tools I've been able to support my clients with. These tools have been acquired through many different experiences. I want to encourage you to value all of your life experiences, to value your innate callings and gifts. They matter just as much, if not more, than any piece of paper you'll ever receive.

PAPER QUALIFICATIONS ARE NOT EVERYTHING

I don't know about you, but in the world I've grown up in, it seems like credentials, degrees, and all kinds of accolades get dangled before us as ultimate prizes. If we're not careful, we may inappropriately bring that mindset into areas of our life. How our minds connect to achievement could possibly be barriers to comprehensive care.

What good is a degree or certificate if you can't listen and connect with the people you serve and support? When we listen in about the Black maternal health crisis, not only in the United States but world-wide, one of the main challenges is that patients, people, and clients are not being listened to. Their complaints are not being heard. They're being dismissed when they share what type of symptoms they're experiencing. Even in the history of gynecological care in the US, when it was first established, it was said that Black women didn't feel pain, so they were experimented on, poked, prodded, and cut open without adequate pain relief and without their consent; and all of this was being done by folks who held degrees and certificates.

So, I want you to walk with me here, as we ponder what our personal connection is, to degrees, credentials, certificates, whatever it is. While it is of the utmost importance to be well-rounded and trained, your certificates, credentials, and degrees do not supersede the level of holistic care you should be able to provide. I want you to answer a couple of these questions before we move forward:

- Does having a degree make you feel like you are the authority in any space you're in?

- Does having a particular credential make you feel you are better than another person?

- Do you rely on your degree to give you permission to not listen to information that is being presented to you in the moment?

If you answered yes to any of those questions, let this be a moment of self-reflection that you take. Have you considered that information, research, and understanding of many different topics is ever evolving, and that there might be a whole host of new information that's been discovered since you received your degree?

When supporting Black families and birth, it is extremely important not to slip into the "savior complex" or any other dismissive role. As a doula supporting Black families, it is important that you understand that you are there to empower, affirm, educate, and advocate. You are there to learn about the people before you and support and affirm them accordingly. While your training and the information you have learned are invaluable assets to your journey overall, they cannot be used to dismiss someone else's literal experiences, background, history, and knowledge of self.

The history of the savior complex, as it relates to Black families, is pervasive in many industries. Whether it is religious colonizing, the history of gynecology, or the wisdom of the grand midwives being co-opted and becoming the foundation of modern-day midwifery in the West, the basis of all of these instances is the following thought. The idea that "I know better than you because I have this credential degree background, and so, now, whether I've gotten the information from you or not, I'm going to feed it back to you, and you have to certify you can jump through this hoop or that hoop to prove to me that you are equal and on par." Which is not always correct.

It's also important to be mindful of prejudices and judgments that we have around credentialing, especially when it comes to communities of different ethnicities. We view credentialing degrees and certificates differently. That is a history lesson for a different day, but I will share this. There are certain communities, particularly Asian or Eurocentric communities, that place an extremely high value on credentialing as a status symbol. Whether the knowledge that was shared and acquired in that credentialing was comprehensive or not, just having that piece of paper is something that is held in high regard. Whereas, lots of other communities, Latino, African, and otherwise, are typically communal by nature and share information, and have shared information historically, via oral tradition. So, there's also the understanding that having a degree, or knowledge from a degree, doesn't make something true, and having something passed down as oral tradition or communal knowledge does not make that information false or inadequate.

THE RIGHT FIT

Body language is 70 to 93 percent of all communication. Why does this matter as it pertains to supporting Black women? This matters because despite how well your intentions are set in supporting a family, if there is anything underneath the surface, ill feelings, judgments, or prejudices that you or anyone around you holds, they will show up in your body language. A smile, accompanied by the right words, does not supersede the strength of nonverbal communication.

When you're showing up to support a Black family, you have to understand that in almost every space we're in, we are accustomed to feeling dislike, hate, and stares, or the energy that we are unwanted in those spaces. We're in tune with it. We know what it looks like, we know what it feels like, and we know what it sounds like, regardless of the words that are being said. We know what the tone of voice sounds like as well.

If you have not done the work and you are not completely honest with yourself, you might find yourself in a very uncomfortable position, both for you and the family that you're seeking to support. Just because you haven't taken the time to become self-aware and reflect on how you're showing up in this space. Note that it's okay to be at a certain point on your journey that says, "Hey, I'm not the best person to support this family."

That actually shows maturity, self-awareness, and thoughtfulness toward the people that you want to see supported. Taking on any family with any background and any values, especially ones that are in direct opposition to ones that you hold or ones that make you uncomfortable, does a disservice to that family and does a disservice to you. So, again, honesty, self-awareness, and reflection are going to be at the core of your birth work practice consistently. This does not just apply to people that have different ethnicities. You could share an ethnicity and have vastly different values such that it would make it uncomfortable for one person or another to be supported by you, and that's okay.

There are enough birthing people to go around, but just as the families are asking for your support as a doula and they're interviewing you to see if you would be a good fit, you're also interviewing them to be a good fit. You're an expert on who you are and what's important to you, and it's essential to be discerning and to understand your capacity to support any family that comes to you seeking your care.

CONFIDENCE MATTERS

How you show up in your space says a lot about your confidence in yourself and your capabilities. This is where trust is built. This is where you can make or break your business. Are you confident in your abilities, or do you feel you haven't had enough practice to execute them properly? Now, this is one of the challenges that my mentees have gone through, and they have confided in me about that challenge over the years. Even after the training, quizzes, tests, and hands-on practice during their weekend trainings, they get thrust into the world and suddenly are frozen, because they don't feel equipped to support a real-life family. Why is that? It's because there's something that they needed to lock into.

It's common for new doulas to feel nervous or uncertain when they first begin their work. One reason for this could be that providing support to families during birth and postpartum is a highly emotional and intense experience. It's natural for anyone new to this type of work to feel overwhelmed or unsure how to handle certain situations. Additionally, every family is unique and has their own set of needs and preferences. Doulas may need to adjust their approach and support methods to best meet the needs of each family they work with. This can require flexibility and adaptability, which can be challenging for someone new to the role. And like with any new job, there is a learning curve involved with becoming a doula. It may take time and practice to build confidence and expertize in supporting families during birth and postpartum.

I know well that new doulas need to build up their conference to serve their clients at a high level. Building confidence as a doula involves several key steps, including:

1. *Experience*: Gain experience by attending births, volunteering at local hospitals, or birthing centers, and working with expectant parents. This will help you develop your skills and gain confidence in your abilities.

2. *Support and mentorship*: Seek out the support of other doulas and mentors who can provide guidance, advice, and encouragement. This can be especially helpful in the early stages of your doula career.

3. *Reflection and evaluation*: Reflect on your experiences as a doula and evaluate your performance. Ask for feedback from clients and other professionals to identify areas where you can improve and build on your strengths.

But what happens when mentees have never attended a birth before? If they believe and tell themselves something like...

- "I can do it. I'm flexible."

- "I can support this family at a high level."

- "I'll pay attention to the details and make it work."

...a confident person will show up in that space knowing that, whether they've attended one birth or one hundred, they are capable of navigating whatever happens. It is just the same as someone who could have attended 50 births but still feels super insecure about their capabilities—your confidence matters.

Make sure you ask questions, team up with a mentor, and have actual opportunities beyond your initial training to build confidence and become confident in who you are as a birth worker. If you walk into a consultation without confidence, it will show all over your face. You may be wondering, "Why hasn't anyone hired me? I don't know what's going on," and it's only going to fuel the negative self-talk that already exists, confirming the doubts that you already have. But I'm here to tell you it's based on your confidence, and your confidence in yourself and your capabilities is what builds trust in your future clients. If confidence is something that you struggle with outside of birth work, that's something to note. Make sure, again, that you are continually developing yourself, and being honest with yourself, so that you know and can identify those areas of improvement.

MAKING CONNECTIONS

Another aspect that can help doulas is understanding the value of heart and spirit connection in service-based professions. So often, people are dismissed, unheard, and even criticized daily. When a family is hiring a doula to support them, they are hoping and praying that you can connect with them, their heart and their desires, and support them fully.

Have you ever been to a massage therapist who had very cold and sterile movements? You could tell that their heart was not in what they were doing. Conversely, have you been to a massage therapist that made you feel like heaven on earth? With each movement and knead, they seemed to be just as joyful and happy to release the pain as you were to feel the discomfort released and tension released from your muscles. That's because their heart and their spirit are in the work that they do.

It is a reality that some doulas may not connect to every client they serve; it doesn't happen for everyone, every time. This could be personality-based or because of some other factor. However, I absolutely believe and teach that we should make that connection as much and as often as possible. Birth work is something that is deeply sacred and spiritual. Therefore, it is important, and it is my belief, that every birth worker needs to seek a heart and spirit connection to the clients and the families that they serve. Your ability to truly connect with your clients will supersede any certificate or degree you obtain. So, take pride in the essence of who you are, and your clients will be attracted to that. The clients that are for you will be attracted to you as you authentically show up in your space.

CHAPTER 4

Deep Nourishment

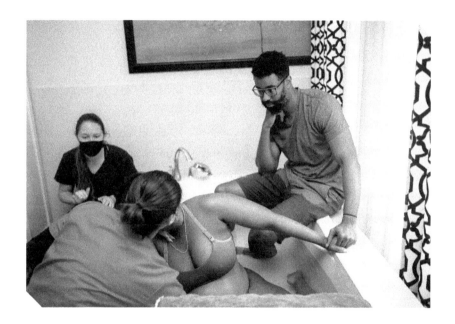

When I moved to Colorado, I was so excited to embark on a new journey in birth work. In Maryland, where I was moving from, home birth was illegal. There were no real birthing centers to speak of, and hospital births were assumed to be the norm. On the East Coast, almost every birth I'd attended was in the hospital. That meant I was accustomed to regular interruptions by nurses and staff, being dismissed as unnecessary, and at times kicked out of my client's rooms.

Out West, home births, birthing centers, and all things crunchy were more of a norm. One winter, I attended the birth of my client's first child at a birth center. At this stage of my birth worker journey, most births I'd attended had been under 24 hours. I foolishly assumed that it would continue to be the case. I attended this birth for over 30 hours, which included a hospital transfer. The air was thick, and the tensions were high due to the changes in the birth plan. A lot of my energy was spent emotionally and spiritually holding space for this couple during the birth of their new baby. By the time their baby made it earthside and everyone had settled in, I grabbed a cup of coffee and headed home. Essentially, I had been away from my family for two days and felt obligated to jump back into the swing of things immediately. My first full day back home wasn't so bad. I was able to go grocery shopping and drop the children off at school just like any other normal day. And then it hit me like a ton of bricks.

On my second day home I came down with one of the worst cases of flu I have ever experienced. Sleep deprivation and lack of good nutrition and hydration left my immune system very vulnerable. I spent the next five days in bed unable to eat, with a fever, muscle aches, and chills. Looking back, it was my lack of experience and naivety that prevented me from preparing my body, my family, and my mind for the possibilities of that birth.

NOURISH YOUR MIND

Continuing to learn about your craft and areas of interest, helps you to be a better birth worker for the clients and families that you support. Being able to nourish your mind with new information, identify and discard old limiting beliefs, and stay abreast on issues as they evolve and change allows you to become well-rounded.

Another reason this is important is that as you continue to be aware of yourself and the thoughts that you're thinking, you can become aware of the blockages that pop up for you as you interact with your clients. This level of awareness is of the utmost importance when it comes to supporting and serving Black women.

Your ability to be aware of your tone, your speech, and making sure that there's no level of dismissiveness or condescension present, is one area that most people ignore when it comes to interacting with historically oppressed groups of people. You may have casual '-isms', and words or phrases that you say that you're very comfortable with, that you may not know are actually very offensive to the group or the individual that you're speaking to. Being able to "read the room" is an extremely beneficial skill set for any birth worker. Whether you're actually in the hospital room, in a home birth space, or even a birth center, being able to feel the tension, read the body language of the folks you are interacting with, as well as a family you're there to support, is of the utmost importance.

Again, I cannot restate enough how important self-awareness is on this journey. Self-awareness not only benefits you, but it literally benefits everyone you come in contact with. When you're able to be aware of the blockages that come up for you, you'll notice that they communicate where growth and healing is still needed. This is an opportunity for personal growth. This is an opportunity for deep nourishment, and this space can shift and change, depending on what phase of life you're actually in.

Here are some ways that deep nourishment of the mind can help you become more self-aware:

- *Cultivating mindfulness*: Mindfulness is the practice of paying attention to the present moment without judgment. By developing this skill, you can become more aware of your thoughts, emotions, and sensations in the moment. This increased awareness can help you to better understand your own inner workings and patterns of behavior.

- *Developing emotional intelligence*: Emotional intelligence refers to the ability to recognize, understand, and manage one's own emotions, as well as the emotions of others. By developing emotional intelligence, you can become more attuned to your own emotional responses and learn to regulate them more effectively.

- *Engaging in self-reflection*: Engaging in regular self-reflection can help you to gain a deeper understanding of your own values, goals, and beliefs. This can help you to identify areas where you may need to make changes in your life, or where you may want to focus your attention.

- *Practicing self-care*: Practicing self-care is an important aspect of mental nourishment. By taking care of your physical and mental health, you can create a strong foundation for introspection and self-awareness. This may include activities such as exercise, meditation, therapy, or simply taking time to relax and recharge.

SET BOUNDARIES

By prioritizing your mental health and well-being, you can create a strong foundation for personal growth and self-discovery. Deep nourishment will demand for you to protect your mind and your heart. In this phase of life, it may be necessary that you're creating stronger boundaries with your family members. Boundaries are necessary to preserve your sense of peace and overall well-being. You must be creating stronger community boundaries, or maybe you're even shifting and showing up in birth work in a new way.

Setting boundaries with family and friends is essential for nurturing overall well-being. It can be challenging to balance personal relationships with the demands of a career that involves being available 24/7. So, here are some steps for approaching setting boundaries with the people closest to you:

1. *Identify your own needs*: Before you can set boundaries with others, it's important to identify your own needs. Reflect on what aspects of your personal life you need to prioritize and protect in order to maintain your overall well-being.

2. *Communicate clearly*: When setting boundaries, it's important to

communicate clearly and assertively with family and friends. Be direct and specific about what you need and why it's important to you.

3. *Be consistent*: Setting boundaries can be challenging, especially with those closest to us. It's important to be consistent in enforcing the boundaries you set, even when it's difficult or uncomfortable.

4. *Offer alternative support*: When setting boundaries with family and friends, it can be helpful to offer alternative sources of support. Let them know that while you may not be available to them at all times, you are still there for them in other ways.

5. *Practice self-care*: Finally, it's important to prioritize self-care when setting boundaries with family and friends. Take time to recharge and nurture your own well-being, and don't be afraid to say no when you need to.

Approaching the people closest to you can be challenging, but it's important to prioritize your own well-being. Consider having an honest and open conversation with them and be clear about what you need in order to maintain balance in your life. Remember that setting boundaries is not about being selfish, but about prioritizing your own well-being so that you can better serve those in your care.

Part of setting boundaries is understanding what you need and where you are headed in your career as a birth worker. Are you considering transitioning to becoming a midwife, or are you continuing your education and going from a certified breastfeeding specialist to a certified lactation consultant (IBCLC)? All of these shifts require different levels of nourishment from your life, from yourself, and from those who support you. It's very important to keep this in mind because all of this will inform your capacity to show up and serve for others, and the only way to do so from a full cup is to make sure that you are deeply nourishing yourself as well, throughout the process of growth.

NOURISH YOUR BODY

Sometimes, we understand that we need to care for ourselves but do not always follow through. It's so easy to become hypocritical when it comes to the suggestions, advocacy, and information that we share with our clients. Oftentimes, we have such a sense of urgency when it comes to talking about the importance of nutrition, exercise, and rest when it comes to pregnant folks that we forget how emotionally, physically, and mentally rigorous birth work can be. But we also need to nourish our bodies in the same way that we're encouraging our clients to.

Taking care of your body is essential to avoid burnout and to be your optimal self within the fieldwork. Here are four ways to take care of your body:

- *Prioritize sleep*: Getting enough sleep is critical for physical and mental health. As a doula, your work may require you to be available at any time of day or night, but it's important to prioritize sleep whenever possible. Make sure to establish a regular sleep schedule and stick to it as much as possible.

- *Practice stress-management techniques*: The work of a doula can be stressful, so it's important to have techniques for managing stress. This may include activities such as meditation, yoga, or deep breathing exercises.

- *Stay hydrated and nourished*: As a doula, you may be on your feet for long periods of time, so it's important to stay hydrated and well-nourished. Make sure to drink plenty of water and eat healthy, nutrient-rich foods to maintain your energy levels throughout the day.

- *Engage in regular physical activity*: Regular physical activity is important for maintaining physical and mental health. As a doula, whilst you'll be more active than in a traditional office job, it's still important to find ways to incorporate physical activity into your daily routine. This could include walking, jogging, or yoga.

AVOID OVERSCHEDULING

A lot of us get into this field because of our own birth experiences or the ones that we've witnessed. This can create an imbalanced desire to take on more than we can handle because of subconscious desires to "fix" or "heal" previous unrelated experiences. It's so important to check in with your body and be clear on what it is you have a capacity to handle. For instance, if you have a lot of younger children at home or you have something else that you are giving and dedicating your time to, it may be important to make sure that you are only taking on one or two birth clients for this season, so that you don't run your body ragged.

Whereas if you're in another season of life, where maybe you're a birth worker that does not have children at all, or your children are older and out of the home, you could possibly increase your capacity to two to three clients, or even two to four clients, as well as traveling in and out of state, but knowing what you actually have a physical capacity for is going to be top priority in this process. You must not overschedule yourself with more than you can handle as this can cause stress and will negatively impact everything in your life, starting with your mental health.

It's important to avoid overscheduling yourself in order to prevent burnout and maintain your physical and mental health. Here are some tips for avoiding overscheduling:

- *Set realistic expectations*: Be honest with yourself about how much time and energy you have available for doula work. Set realistic expectations for the number of clients you can take on at any given time.

- *Prioritize self-care*: Make self-care a priority in your life, and schedule time for activities that help you relax and recharge. This may include things like exercise, spending time in nature, or spending time with loved ones.

- *Learn to say no*: It can be difficult to turn down potential clients, but it's important to know when to say no. If you feel that you are already at capacity, or if taking on another client would cause you to overschedule yourself, it's okay to decline the opportunity.

- *Use a scheduling system*: Use a scheduling system to help you manage your time effectively. This may include tools such as a calendar, scheduling app, or task manager. Make sure to build in time for breaks and downtime to prevent overscheduling.

- *Create boundaries*: Set boundaries with clients to ensure that you are not overextending yourself. This may include establishing clear communication channels, setting expectations around response times, and scheduling regular check-ins to ensure that everyone is on the same page.

Remember that supporting families will require your strength and energy. How can you provide the proper support to your clients if you are feeling exhausted and depleted? On the other hand, how can you care for your own family if you are stressed and feel overworked? Pushing yourself to the max is never good.

PREPARE YOURSELF

Nourishing your body deeply is extremely important for preparing you to support a family during birth. You want to make sure that you have the energy, the nutrients, and the stamina to support your family at full capacity. What does that look like? That looks like making sure that you are consistently hydrated. It looks like making sure that you know what vitamins and minerals you need for your body to be in balance and taking them on a consistent basis. It also looks like getting adequate rest as you're preparing for the birth support.

In my experience, I begin to prepare for each birth about a week or two in advance. I begin making sure that I'm getting sleep on a consistent basis, that I'm going to bed on time. I also make sure that I'm getting a consistent flow of nutritious food, so that my body is not starting from zero when my client randomly goes into birth. It also looks like, on a consistent level, making sure that I'm aware of my hormone levels and how they're impacting my energy, my strength, and my ability to perform.

LOOK AFTER YOURSELF

Now, I want to make a note here. Being a birth worker is a very nurturing and caring career path. Often with caregivers, you will find that they neglect their own personal health to serve and support their communities, their families, and their loved ones. This is something that is actually, ultimately, to the detriment of the people that they say they care about. If we are not serving from a full cup and we're unable to show up whole, healthy, and strong, we're not going to be around as long as we think we will. For most of us, I'm sure that's not what we desire; but as a birth worker, if you would like to see any type of longevity in this work, and on this path, it's very important that you take care of your body, your mind, and your spirit. As you know, supporting a family and birth can be very physically rigorous, so not only must you ensure that your body is strong, your mind is sound, and your heart is grounded, you also have to make sure that on a very practical level, you know where you stand.

Heart-centered work is very draining. It is draining on the mind, it's draining on the heart and it's draining on the spirit; but more importantly, it's extremely draining (can be very taxing) on the body. I cannot stress enough how important it is to make sure that you yourself are getting your hormone levels checked, and you yourself are aware of any diseases or conditions that you have that might require adaptation in how you're able to support others.

I cannot overstate how important it is to know your own needs for mental and physical nourishment so that you are able to support and serve at the highest level, without breaking your body down when it comes to supporting others. Your family needs you. They want you to be around for a while. Your community needs you. They would love to see you love and serve and support them for as long as you are able or desire to; but most importantly, you need you, and it's so important to keep you front of mind, your physical health front of mind, as you are embarking on this journey.

I alluded to this previously, but support is best given from a full cup. It's important that we let the overflow of our heart be the space that we serve and support our families from. A lot of us don't even know what serving from a full cup feels like, and sadly, that's a shame; but it's important that we are diligent in doing the self-work, where we discover what service from a full cup actually is and remain committed to it.

What does this look like? For some, it may look like taking a break from birth work if your own life requires your full attention and energy. For others, it looks like working in areas of birth work that have a set schedule that is easy to adjust and fit in with their personal and family life schedule. For others, this simply looks like being aware of the ebbs and flows of their personal lives and creating strong boundaries with their loved ones, their clients, and their community, so that they have time to nourish themselves the way that they need to be nourished.

Don't allow social media to thrust you into spaces you are not emotionally or spiritually prepared for. If you are still processing different traumas that are related to birth, I cannot stress this enough. It is of the utmost importance that you address any birth trauma that you have or any birth trauma that you have witnessed. It is of my personal perspective and belief that therapy of some form needs to be a part of every birth worker's tool bag. Making sure that you're consistently keeping a clean and clear palette with regard to the trauma that you've witnessed is something that you do, not only for your clients, but for yourself.

Healing from trauma related to birth experiences can be a complex and deeply personal process. Here are some strategies that may be helpful:

- *Seek professional support*: Consider seeking the support of a mental health professional with experience in trauma and perinatal mental health. A trained therapist can help you work through your feelings and emotions in a safe and supportive environment.

- *Join a support group*: Connecting with others who have experienced similar trauma can be validating and supportive. Look for support groups or online communities focused on perinatal mental health and birth trauma.

- *Practice self-care*: Make self-care a priority in your life. This may include activities such as exercise, meditation, spending time in nature, or spending time with loved ones.

- *Consider alternative therapies*: Alternative therapies such as acupuncture, massage, or yoga may be helpful in reducing stress and anxiety related to birth trauma.

- *Educate yourself*: Educate yourself on the experiences of birth trauma and how it can impact mental health. This can help you gain a better understanding of your own experiences and feelings.

- *Give yourself time*: Healing from trauma is a process that takes time. Be patient with yourself and allow yourself the space and time needed to heal.

It's important to note that healing from birth trauma is a deeply personal process, and what works for one person may not work for another. If you are struggling with trauma related to a birth experience, consider reaching out for support and exploring a range of strategies to find what works best for you. Continuing to heal, grow, and love takes work and consistency. It's not something that happens overnight, it happens because you desire it. It takes intentionality. It takes support. It takes time, but it's one of the ways that you will burn out the quickest if it's not addressed and taken care of properly.

CHAPTER 5

Everything Is Connected

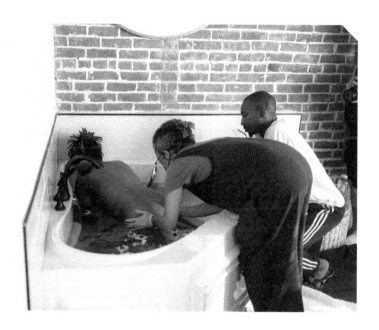

Copal filled the room, and the lingering sound of native lullabies rang in our ears. The smell of beans and rice, chicken and corn, and body fluids, wafted through the air as we waited. We danced. They slept. The elders laughed downstairs recounting stories of their own in anticipation of the one being written. With each click-clack of her Flamenco shoes, the memories shook from deep within her. I remember the moment I saw her face change. She was no longer present. No longer the fiery, birthing woman preparing to birth her legacy. As she began weeping, it became clear that the pain she was experiencing had nothing to do with her contractions. It was emotional, it was deep, it was personal. Birth is unpredictable like that. You never know which experiences will be shaken loose to reveal themselves at the most inopportune moments. Holding space for what was, in grieving what is, was what the moment called for. There's no way we could have prepared for that in any prenatal consult, and I'm not sure that we should have. Holding space while someone gives birth is sacred. It's sacred for the moment it is, it's sacred for the moment to come, and it's sacred because in those moments we get a chance to ride the nuanced waves of the humanity of another person.

As you are supporting Black women and other women of color, it's important to keep top of mind the understanding of how everything is connected. In neuroscience, there is an understanding that the soul, growth and mental strength, behavior, capacity, and environment are all linked together. Your past experiences, emotions, and how you've processed them may be activated in current circumstances that feel familiar to your brain. These memories can be from childhood, adolescence, or even adulthood. Self-awareness helps you discern, in each moment, how your body, mind, and spirit are reacting or interacting with your clients, their providers, and your surroundings.

When trauma or flashbacks of similar experiences show up in your body, it has the potential to freeze your mind and impair your decision-making. What does that look like when you're supporting a birth? If you have unidentified prejudices and judgments against people of color, or maybe you were even raised to have certain beliefs about different communities, this may show up in moments that you wouldn't expect. Even if you've gone the majority of your life having the Black friend or the Latino hair stylist, and you feel that you were able to interact in a very healthy way with them, without that level of self-awareness in play, you will not be able to identify those subconscious judgments.

The birthing space is so open, and so vulnerable and so intense, that it often causes many emotions to rise to the surface for your clients, but it also can have many emotions and feelings arise for you. It's an emotionally charged experience. It's important to have strategies in place to cope with moments of vulnerability and maintain your own emotional well-being. Here are some tips for coping with vulnerability during a birth:

- *Practice self-awareness*: Be aware of your own emotions and reactions during the birth experience. Take time to reflect on your own feelings and thoughts and acknowledge them without judgment.

- *Focus on your breathing*: When you feel overwhelmed or vulnerable, focus on your breathing. Take deep, slow breaths, and visualize yourself exhaling tension and anxiety.

- *Use positive affirmations*: Use positive affirmations to help you stay grounded and focused. Repeat phrases such as "I am calm and centered" or "I am a source of support and comfort."

- *Connect with your client*: Stay connected with your client throughout the birth process. Offer words of encouragement and validation and remind them that they are strong and capable.

- *Take breaks*: If you feel overwhelmed or need a moment to regroup, take a break. Step out of the room for a few minutes, get some fresh air, and take a few deep breaths.

It's so important, so, so important, to be self-aware and in tune with your body, so that as these feelings and these judgments arise, you can stick a pin in them and adjust them later, or be able to push them aside, so that you can focus on your client in the moment. Example: If you have a subconscious belief, as many do, that Black women don't feel pain the same as other people, when your client is expressing discomfort, you could find yourself not believing them, because you have a subconscious prejudice that is backed by old science. There is this belief that Black people don't experience pain, or they experience pain on a significantly decreased level than other ethnicities. When it comes time to support your client, your ability to show up wholly, fully, and be able to believe what they say they're experiencing, is where those beliefs will show up.

If you believe that your client is overreacting, or if you believe that they're making things out to be more than what they are, you will be less likely to support them and respond to their needs appropriately. Just because you're a birth worker does not mean that you are incapable of having the same dismissive, problematic perspectives that are consistently attributed to systematic Western healthcare. We all have judgments and preconceived notions that we come to the table with, and it is always important to understand how they're linked together, how they show up, how we interact with others, and even present in our career paths.

Self-awareness helps you discern, in each moment, how your body, mind, and spirit are reacting or interacting with your clients, their providers, and your surroundings. When trauma or flashbacks of similar experiences show up in our bodies, it has the potential to freeze our minds and impair our decision-making. When your client is in the middle of needing your support, or if you are engaging with them through conversation or maybe even virtual support, it's so important to be aware that you are showing up fully. You must show up in the identity that you know you desire to have and be as a birth worker.

When you have experienced trauma, inevitably there are triggers—and you must be aware of your triggers. But how can you be aware and be able to anticipate them if you don't know what they are. First, let's talk about what triggers are. What are triggers? Triggers derived from trauma are experiences or situations that can elicit a strong emotional or physical response in someone who has experienced the trauma. These triggers can be anything that reminds the person of the traumatic event, such as a sound, smell, or image, and can lead to feelings of anxiety, fear, anger, or sadness.

To identify if what you are feeling is a trigger, it can be helpful to pay attention to your body's reactions to certain situations or experiences. Some common physical reactions to triggers include increased heart rate, sweating, shaking, and feeling lightheaded or dizzy. Emotional reactions can include feeling overwhelmed, anxious, sad, angry, or numb.

If you notice that you are experiencing these physical or emotional reactions in response to certain situations or experiences, it may be helpful to explore whether these reactions are related to a past trauma. Speaking with a mental health professional can help you identify triggers and develop coping strategies to manage their effects.

It's difficult to deal with triggers in moments where birth work requires you to be all-in emotionally, spiritually, and mentally. Are you compassionate? Are you nurturing? Are you remaining objective? Guess what? We all have moments where we are not as objective as some might like us to be, and sometimes that is beneficial, and sometimes it's not.

Here's an example. If I'm supporting a family who is used to interacting with hospital staff in a particular way—maybe they're not as educated on the terminology and the words used—they just blindly trust the hospital staff. In such a scenario, I could remain neutral and say, "Well, as long as they're okay with it, I'm okay with it," or I could put on my advocacy hat and make sure that I am very clearly spelling out, in layman's terms, what is being communicated to my client for them to understand what their choices are moving forward.

I can also see the coercion taking place in the birthing space more quickly than that family because I witness more often. Now, we don't have to become hyper-vigilant, aggressive, or anything like that, but, as a birth worker, it's easier for me to discern:

- what's happening or what's about to transpire

- when something isn't being communicated honestly

- why something is harmful

- why something can be helpful.

As a doula, I can communicate clearly with my clients what's happening at any moment so that they can fully understand the situation or experience. The goal is to make sure our clients are truly receiving correct information about everything that they're experiencing, and that everything they're being told is clear to them. This is key. Everything is connected. Understanding how things are intertwined can help you become a well-rounded doula. You must develop the proper communication skills and learn to navigate tough situations. Developing and improving spiritual connections with others while also nurturing yourself is essential.

As you walk your birth worker journey, seek to grow, and learn as much as possible about responding to different situations. All birth experiences are different. They are unpredictable, and you never know what will happen. Things can take a turn for the worse quickly, and you need to act appropriately, instead of responding with a flight or fight reaction.

If you have had a natural birth experience, you know that the woman giving birth goes through many waves of emotions. There is uncertainty and fear, especially when they are vividly experiencing every wave of contractions as they come and go. Contractions become intense, and sometimes women can be in control, whereas others feel like giving up because they feel like the pain is too much to bear.

In the middle of a birthing experience, you don't only have to support the woman giving birth but also guide the people around her at that moment. Sometimes the spouse is nervous or can get worried, so you also have to deal with those emotions and provide support, compassion, empathy, and reassurance.

The entire birthing journey is an emotionally charged experience for many people who are involved in it. Thus, it's important for you to develop emotional intelligence. It involves being able to identify and express emotions appropriately, regulate one's own emotions, empathize with others, and handle interpersonal relationships effectively.

Being emotionally intelligent is vital for several reasons. First, it can help individuals better understand their feelings and motivations, leading to increased self-awareness and better decision-making. Second, emotionally intelligent individuals are often better at managing stress and coping with adversity. Third, being emotionally intelligent can help individuals to build stronger relationships with others, both personally and professionally. Finally, studies have shown that emotionally intelligent people tend to be more successful in their careers, as they are better at navigating complex social situations and understanding the needs and motivations of others.[1, 2]

Overall, emotional intelligence is essential to personal and professional development and can significantly impact one's success and well-being. As a support person during the birthing experience, a doula can benefit greatly from being emotionally intelligent. Here are some ways in which emotional intelligence can be helpful for doulas:

- *Understanding and empathizing with the mother's emotions*: Emotional intelligence can help doulas to understand and empathize with the mother's emotional state during labor and delivery. This can allow them to provide emotional support that is tailored to the mother's needs and preferences.

- *Recognizing and managing their own emotions*: Doulas who are emotionally intelligent are better equipped to manage their own emotions during the birthing experience. This can help them remain calm and focused, even in stressful or challenging situations.

- *Building strong relationships with clients*: Emotional intelligence can help doulas to build strong, supportive relationships with their clients. This can lead to better communication, increased trust, and a more positive birthing experience for both the mother and the doula.

- *Navigating complex social dynamics*: Emotional intelligence can help doulas to navigate complex social dynamics that may arise during the birthing experience. For example, they may need to communicate effectively with medical professionals or family members who have different perspectives or goals for the birth.

Emotional intelligence can be a valuable asset for doulas, allowing them to effectively support mothers during the birthing experience.

Let's put things into perspective. There may be a family you're supporting with a history of being in the hospital space, and maybe they're choosing a different route—to give birth in the hospital or at home. It's so important to be able to communicate all of the challenges, all of the benefits, and all of the support that the family will need, to achieve the birth that they desire. It's equally important to encourage them to understand that having flexibility in their birth plan and mentally being able to pivot, if needed, gives them the healthiest outcome possible.

These are just a couple of ways that show how our experiences, our environment, our past, our history, and our culture are all intertwined in how we show up in different spaces. Again, all ethnicities do not have the same cultural experience. Do not feel like you read a book about Black people, and now you get it. Do not think that you spent five years being best friends with a person, and now, you understand their struggle. While you may have an intimate look into a culture, a person's experience, or the experience of a particular family, it's imperative that you keep an open mind. You must understand that not every person shares the same cultural experience. This brings me to inform you of the importance of developing cultural competence.

Being culturally competent and aware of cultural differences is important when communicating with expectant and new parents. This means understanding and respecting different cultural practices and beliefs and adapting your communication style to meet the individual needs of each parent.

There is power in understanding that you need to be open and remain flexible to understand the family and the person that is right in front of you—remaining flexible and open to understanding yourself, and what you're bringing to the table, so that you'll know how to interact powerfully to empower, affirm, and support the family that you're advocating for.

Communication is your primary foundation for building trust and a connection with the birthing mother and her family. It's important to communicate clearly and effectively to ensure that expectations and needs are understood by all parties. This includes setting clear boundaries and expectations and communicating any changes or updates in a timely manner. Using respectful language and avoiding judgmental statements is crucial when communicating with expectant and new parents. This can help build trust and a positive rapport with them. Keep in mind that you will be working with expectant and new parents during a vulnerable and emotional time. It's important to approach communication with empathy and understanding, acknowledging the challenges they may be facing. And along with empathy is an important pillar of communication that will help you serve your families with excellence—active listening.

Serving others well is impossible if you are not listening attentively to them. Active listening is one of the most important aspects of communication. This means giving your full attention to the person speaking and taking the time to understand their perspective and concerns. No matter where you find yourself in your journey, seek to improve and ask for feedback from the families that you assist. That way, you receive insight into what you are doing well and what you need to improve.

As a doula, you can inspire, encourage, and fully support expecting mothers and be part of incredible birth experiences. There is much work to be done. Though you will face challenges, don't give up. Being a birth worker is more than a title or business. It's a divine calling because you play an important role in bringing another human being into this world. The work you do is beyond priceless!

NOTES

1   Urquijo, I., Extremera, N., and Azanza, G. (2019) "The contribution of emotional intelligence to career success: Beyond personality traits." *International Journal of Environmental Research and Public Health* 16, 23, 4809.

2   Pirsoul, T., Parmentier, M., Sovet, L., and Nils, F. (2023) "Emotional intelligence and career-related outcomes: A meta-analysis." *Human Resource Management Review* 33, 3, 100967.

CHAPTER 6

Birthy Biz Structures

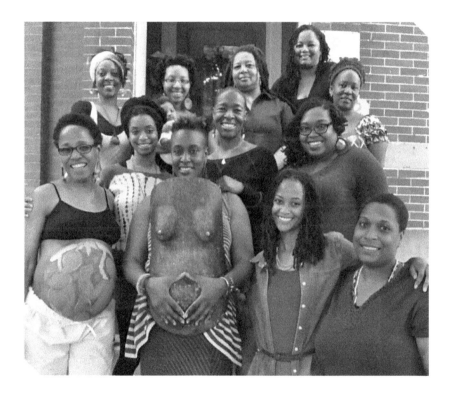

How you structure your birth business is a vital part of your success. There are many different ways to approach your birth business structure. They include:

- community-based birth work
- solo model ("solopreneur")

- agency model

- digital content/product creator.

The most organic and common way of structuring your birth work activity is to become a community-based birth worker. Many community-based birth workers are not necessarily established as a business, but they show up in the community along their pathway. Typically, they serve low- to middle-income demographics, and their practices are full of connection, integrity, reasonable pricing, and even bartering.

There is a high level of connection with grassroots organizations that are super tied in with local organizations, schools, and family networks. Community-based birth work is the most organic, natural type of birth work. By being in community with others, you naturally find what you need by word of mouth. For instance, in your group of friends, there may be an accountant or lawyer and someone else you know looking for an accountant or lawyer, who can be introduced; in a similar way, you can get your referrals within the network of families you surround yourself with.

In the past, and historically speaking, birth workers supported the people in their local town and maybe the towns one or two over. This meant everyone knew whom to call when they needed a midwife and doula. So, back in the day, it would not have been called a "doula," but the midwife's assistants that helped to support the birthing process. And typically, for women in the family, it was expected that they would support one another when it came to time for birth.

When you are a community-based birth worker, there may very well be a cap on how many clients you can support per month. But you also have the benefit of a high level of collaboration with other community-based birth workers, where you guys can support one another, and you have the benefit of familiarity already with the families in your network and any of the other community-based birth workers you would collaborate with.

The next model is the solo model, where a birth worker may establish an LLC or an Inc. This structure operates best when you have a backup doula, maybe even a partner, solid systems, standard operating procedures, and partnerships with local OB-GYN and midwifery offices. Typically, you will also find that there is a cap on clients per month that you're able to take on just because of your physical capacity.

The next model is the agency model, which can be established as an LLC, Inc., etc. One of the capstones of the agency model, or developing an agency model, is leadership, integrity, systems, scheduling, and deciding whether you will run it co-op style, and whether it will be a national or local agency. Agencies are chock-full of resources, as is every other structure. Your cap is typically based on your staff, the amount of staff you have, and their availability.

The last structure is digital. In this new day and age, there is tons of space for people to become digital and/or virtual birth workers. That could mean being a content creator, where you create content centered around different "birthy" topics. It could mean that you create digital products for people to purchase without necessarily interacting with you. That could also mean that you have a heavy presence on social media, where you connect with people, give advice, and book consults on a virtual level. It could also mean that you're an influencer, where you may very well have the reach or the capacity to influence tons of people, and you choose to do so through the demographic of expectant families. There's no cap on the families you can reach in the digital space because technology is expanding daily. New ways, new apps, and new communities are developed to help you expand in many different ways. Thus, using and leveraging those media to help, inform, and reach families considering natural births would be wise.

No matter what model you choose to pursue, it must be a decision that you make from the heart. Your spirit and heart need to be in it. A birthing business is more than a business. It's a calling to bring life into this world. And that is no easy assignment.

Studies show that doulas share common traits—they are compassionate and empathetic.[1] While this is true, your empathy, compassion, and understanding towards your clients may not be helpful to you when it comes to building out your business.

93

As doulas, we have a passion for helping women and their families through one of the most significant experiences of their lives. It's sensitive and emotionally moving. The reality is that doulas work long hours, often including nights and weekends, and must be on call for their clients for weeks before and after the due date. They also often work independently and may face challenges such as navigating medical systems and advocating for their client's wishes. It's a demanding profession in every way.

Therefore, having a genuine passion for supporting and empowering expectant mothers and their families will keep you motivated and committed to your clients and their needs. It's important to note that while passion is necessary, commitment to your journey is also needed because you will face moments of self-doubt.

Self-doubt is a common experience for many doulas and can arise from various factors, such as lack of experience, challenging birth experiences, or difficulties in interpersonal dynamics with clients. Here are some strategies that doulas can use to overcome self-doubt:

- *Seek support*: Doulas can seek support from colleagues, mentors, or other professionals in their network to discuss their doubts, share experiences, and seek guidance.

- *Reflect on past successes*: Doulas can reflect on past successes and remind themselves of their positive impact on their client's lives. This can help them regain confidence in their abilities.

- *Continue learning*: Doulas can seek out continuing education opportunities, attend workshops, or pursue certification in related areas, which can enhance their knowledge, skills, and confidence.

- *Practice self-care*: Doulas can practice self-care, such as getting enough rest, engaging in physical activity, and taking breaks from work to prevent burnout and promote their well-being.

- *Communicate with clients*: Doulas can communicate with their clients about their doubts or concerns, which can help build trust and deepen the relationship. Additionally, talking through client concerns can help the doula feel more confident in their ability to support the client effectively.

It's important to remember that self-doubt is a normal part of any profession, and taking proactive steps to address doubts can help build confidence and improve client outcomes. And your overall experience amid your journey as a birth worker.

NOTES

1   Hansard, K. (2012) "Compassion and empathy—a doula's best friends." *Midwifery Today with International Midwife*. Spring (101), 31, 69.

CHAPTER 7

Spiritual Grounding

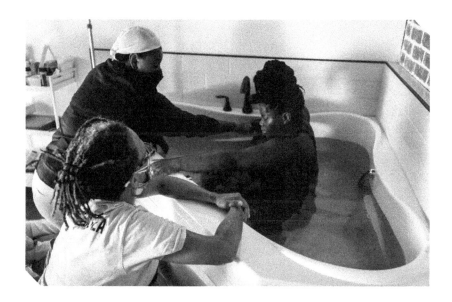

One of my favorite things to do after a birth is turning up my favorite salsa playlist, dancing in my living room, enjoying a comfort meal, and then running a warm bath to relax. Whether a birth has gone exactly as planned or there were some bumps in the road, I need to discharge the energy from my body. Dancing is a way to literally move energy around in your body. Being a part of someone's once-in-a-lifetime experience is not something to take lightly. Even if someone has given birth before, this is their first time giving birth to that baby or having that birth experience. That reality should be honored.

Music is another way I ground myself in preparation and after a birth. On the way in, I typically play music that is very peaceful, calming, and meditative. This allows me the space and time to clear out my own junk before supporting my clients and their families. After a birth, turning up my favorite song and belting out the words on the way home helps ensure I stay awake long enough to make it home safely. It seems so simple, but it's an easy way to trick your brain, especially if you're exhausted.

Your grounding process is going to be tailor-fit to you. There is no right way to do it, but it is always necessary for balance.

MEDITATION

Meditation, as a consistent practice, helps to build self-awareness, to decrease stress, and to ground you. Sitting in silence, or even doing a walking meditation, allows the things that are deep within you to arise for you to see, focus on, and address. Also, in other spiritual practices, meditation can be a time that is used to meditate on verses and phrases that allow you to connect to the Creator. Whatever path you're on, being still, getting aware, and tapping in will remain an amazing tool for you as a birth worker. If you've had a rough day, gotten cut off fifty-eleven times on the highway, and are now headed into a birth, you might be a little frazzled, a little on edge, and possibly agitated. But the family you are preparing to support deserves to have the clearest, calmest, and most centered version of you. That way, you're ready to observe, advocate, affirm, and encourage them from the most grounded, clearest space possible.

It may seem counter-intuitive, but you need to flip the switch before entering the space and supporting the family during the birth and postpartum. Meditation is a tool that is very helpful in bringing you back to the center. Meditation can be helpful in several ways. Here are a few benefits of meditation practice:

- *Reduces stress and anxiety*: Meditation is known to have a calming effect on the mind, which can help reduce stress and anxiety.

- *Improves focus and concentration*: Regular meditation practice can improve your ability to focus and concentrate. It helps to train your mind to stay in the present moment.

- *Enhances emotional well-being*: Meditation can help you develop greater self-awareness and self-acceptance. It helps to cultivate positive emotions like compassion and empathy.

- *Lowers blood pressure*: Studies have shown that regular meditation practice can help lower blood pressure and reduce the risk of heart disease.[1]

- *Improves sleep*: Meditation can help to calm the mind and relax the body, making it easier to fall asleep and stay asleep.

- *Boosts the immune system*: Regular meditation practice has been shown to boost the immune system, which can help protect against illness and disease.

Meditation can help promote physical, mental, and emotional well-being, making it a valuable tool for anyone looking to improve their overall health and quality of life. So, you can imagine how helpful it is for you as a birth worker and how you can recommend it to birthing mothers.

PRAYER

Another practice that is beneficial is prayer. You can process any emotion or any experience through the power of prayer. Prayer is an amazingly comforting, grounding process. It's a beautiful way for you to connect with the Creator and allow yourself to speak and open up about what you may be enduring. Prayer can help you heal and go through your challenges. When you have faith, you have hope. Hope is a powerful emotion.

For some, prayer is utilized as a covering during the birth experience. Depending on their beliefs, prayer is a way to connect to the family you're supporting. Likewise, coming out of the birth experience, prayer is sometimes utilized to give thanks for the experience that was just had and provide blessings for the family as they move into their postpartum season.

THERAPY

Another avenue to find grounding is through therapy. You can find a therapist to talk to or somatic therapy. Another form of therapy that is effective is group therapy. No matter what you choose, they are all amazing ways to process your inner world of emotions. If you have experienced trauma, seeking therapy of any kind will be extremely helpful, whether it's before or after helping the family with their birthing experience. Therapy is beneficial for all parties involved in the birthing process.

I'm not suggesting that as soon as you depart from the family after birth, you are going through this rigorous process of discharging everything you've experienced. But it is helpful to talk and process your emotions tied to the birthing experience. For some, it may take you days or even weeks to realize how that birth experience is settling in your body, settling in your mind or maybe even triggering something in you, positive or negative, that is now resonating with you weeks after.

As doulas, we provide emotional and physical support to women and their partners during childbirth, and we often develop close relationships with our clients. Witnessing a difficult or traumatic birth can be emotionally challenging for a doula, especially if the experience triggers their own past traumas or feelings of helplessness.

Some common experiences that can be traumatic for doulas include witnessing a long or difficult labor, witnessing medical interventions that were not desired by the mother, witnessing the loss of a baby, or feeling powerless to help the mother or baby during a complication. We need to take care of our own emotional and mental health and seek support if we experience trauma from a birthing experience.

As mentioned previously, this may include talking to a therapist or counselor, debriefing with other birth professionals, or taking time off to process our emotions. When you take care of yourself, you can continue to provide compassionate care to your clients in the future. Therapy is a beautiful way to process your feelings in an objective environment. Somatic therapy is an amazing way to move the trauma, or secondary trauma, through and out of your body so that you can understand and operate from your own baseline. Somatic therapy is a type of therapy that focuses on the mind–body connection. It can help you identify and release physical sensations associated with emotions, such as tension, pain, or discomfort. Somatic therapy may involve movement, touch, or other techniques to help you process emotions at a physical level.

BEING PHYSICALLY PREPARED

In preparation for birth, movement is so important. Making sure that you have a regular exercise regimen is going to be something that is extremely helpful for you on your birth journey. Making sure that your body is stretched out and limber is going to be of the utmost importance. Making sure that you are getting cardio in, on a regular basis, helps with your cardiovascular system. You will make sure that your heart is strong, but before every birth, I'm here to tell you, you never know what to expect. So, stretching is going to be your best friend.

Making sure that you have good/optimum nutrition in preparation for birth support is also a wise decision. Ensuring you have vitamins, alkaline water, good grains, healthy proteins, and even a splash of chlorophyll in your water can go a long way in ensuring that you are grounded and ready to support this upcoming birth.

A huge part of your health is your sleep routine. There's no quicker way to be scatterbrained and feeling not like yourself than to operate from sleep deprivation. As I mentioned earlier in Chapter 4, one of the ways that I prepare for birth support is by making sure that I'm intentionally getting tons of rest. This is especially important as I'm approaching my client's due date.

The anticipation is high in the couple of weeks leading up to the baby's arrival. The phone ringer is turned all the way up, and the alarms are preset. Because of that, you may find yourself having difficulty getting sleep. This might mean that if you're unable to get rest at night as you usually do, you prepare and get naps in during the day. You need to help your body to get the rest and recharge it needs and deserves.

The other thing is that you must get the rest you need after attending a birth. In my experience, I've seen myself take anywhere between one full day to five full days to recover from a birth. This definitely depends on the level of physical engagement that took place at the time a woman gave birth. It depends on how emotionally taxing it was. It also is contingent upon how well-nourished I was physically, emotionally, and mentally before entering that space. So, these are all things to consider when discussing making sure you are spiritually grounded.

JOURNALING

Another helpful practice on your birth work journey and business is journaling. Journaling may also be your best friend. It is a way to write out and process your thoughts and emotions, especially after having attended a birth journey. Journaling can offer many benefits for mental health and well-being. Here are two benefits of journaling:

- *Reduces stress and anxiety*: Writing about your thoughts, feelings, and experiences in a journal can help reduce stress and anxiety. By putting your thoughts on paper, you may find that you can let go of some of the thoughts that are causing you stress. Additionally, journaling can help you gain perspective on a situation, which can reduce anxiety.

- *Increases self-awareness and self-reflection*: Journaling can help you become more self-aware by giving you a space to reflect on your thoughts and experiences. By taking time to write down your thoughts, you may gain insight into your feelings and behaviors. You may also be able to identify patterns in your thinking or behavior that you want to change. Overall, journaling can help you develop a better understanding of yourself, which can lead to personal growth and increased self-confidence.

Intentionally reflecting on what you just witnessed and being able to itemize it on paper, look at it and reflect on it later will become something of great value to you in the future.

Overall, engaging in self-nourishing practices, such as praying, sitting in silence, and acknowledging if anything came up for you during birth support, is of the utmost importance. Reflecting on whether there is any residue from previous traumas you've experienced or if there's any way you could have shown up better is always something beautiful to reflect on. Leaning into your restoration and refilling your cup is a beautiful practice. And although it may not always be easy, it is worth it. And this does not only apply in birth work but in every area of your life.

As we have seen, the work of a doula is a beautiful and meaningful profession that can bring great fulfillment and satisfaction. Doulas play a vital role in helping families have positive and empowering birth experiences by providing emotional and physical support to women and their partners during childbirth. To be most successful and fulfilled as a doula, it's important to prioritize self-care and maintain healthy boundaries with clients. This includes taking time off to recharge, seeking support from other birth professionals, and being mindful of your own emotional and mental well-being. By taking care of yourself, you can continue to provide compassionate and effective care to your clients and positively impact the world of birth work. When choosing to walk the path of supporting others deeply during vulnerable moments in life, it is good spiritual hygiene to refresh, reset, and nourish yourself. This spiritual grounding is an integral part of our lives both as doulas and as humans.

NOTES

1   Harvard Health Publishing (2023, July 18) "Meditation and a relaxation technique to lower blood pressure." www.health.harvard.edu/heart-health/meditation-and-a-relaxation-technique-to-lower-blood-pressure

CHAPTER 8

Pregnancy Loss and Its Impact on You

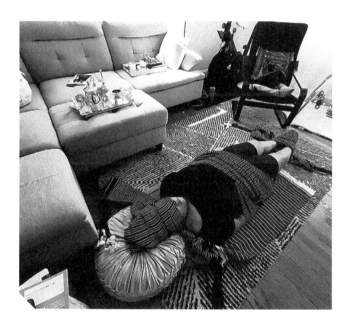

I remember the call like it was yesterday. A long-time birth client reached out to let me know that their newest addition didn't make it. My heart sank. Every celebratory call and conversation we'd had over the last couple of months flashed quickly before my eyes. The moments of euphoria and joy we felt during the previous births started to fade in my mind. As I felt my heart beating through my chest, I reminded myself to breathe. Just breathe.

As the tears fell, I searched for words to comfort her, somehow, someway. Grasping for words like we grasp for air when we've been underwater just a few seconds too long, I couldn't find them. I felt helpless, overwhelmed with emotion, and instantly exhausted. This was the moment I knew my sabbatical from birth support would be longer than expected.

The last four years or so have been riddled with an unmatched level of collective and personal grief and trauma for most people in the world. Loss after loss has been shared on social media, family group chats, and within our friend circles. The birthing space is no different. As humans, we aren't designed to process so much information and emotions in a short span of time. Quite frankly, it's been consistently overwhelming... I don't know what else to say.

Trauma is a personal experience. What might be traumatizing for one person may not be traumatizing for another. The ability to hear, listen to, and discern when someone is expressing a traumatic experience is critical to helping you figure out where to allocate support.

DIFFERENT TYPES OF TRAUMA

There are different types of trauma—personal, familial, collective, and workplace trauma, as well as secondary trauma. Understanding the nuances and difference between these is very helpful. Let's have an in-depth look at what each type of trauma means and its impact on individuals and beyond.

- *Personal trauma*: Think of personal trauma as an experience that happens to a person causing them physical or psychological pain and harm. A personal trauma can be the result of an incident, such as an accident, a natural disaster, personal loss, or death of a loved one. Personal traumas are rooted in experiences like childhood abuse, neglect, or witnessing violence (secondary trauma). The impact of personal trauma can include symptoms of depression, anxiety, flashbacks, and nightmares, among others.

- *Familial trauma*: Familial trauma refers to traumatic experiences that affect an entire family or multiple generations within a family. This type of trauma can be passed down from generation to generation—it's intergenerational. For instance, a familial trauma can be dysfunction in the family, such as a history of violence, domestic abuse, or unresolved family secrets. If there is familial trauma within a family unit, there is possible lack of communication or recurring patterns of behavior that perpetuate the trauma's impact.

- *Collective trauma*: Collective trauma affects an entire community, society, or group of people. It occurs on a large scale. We see collective trauma in communities or countries that have experienced war, terrorist attacks, pandemics, or natural disasters. Unfortunately, collective trauma can have far-reaching consequences leading to a shared sense of grief and loss. We can look back and know that we all suffered collective trauma at different levels because of the Covid-19 pandemic. The impact of collective trauma is the feeling of being vulnerable, afraid, and having to rebuild a sense of security. It takes time for communities to recover.

- *Workplace trauma*: Then we have workplace trauma. It encompasses traumatic experiences in one's job or in the work environment. This type of trauma can be a result of experiencing discrimination of any sort, exposure to distressing events, physical violence, or harassment. This kind of trauma can have lasting effects on a person's mental health and emotional well-being.

- *Secondary trauma*: Secondary trauma, often referred to as vicarious trauma, is a type of trauma that happens when a person is an exposed to the traumatic experiences of the suffering of another person rather than experiencing the trauma firsthand. The key characteristics of secondary trauma are as follows: indirect exposure, empathic response, physical and emotional symptoms, professional context, and cumulative effect. Indirect exposure happens when someone is exposed to and is a witness to the trauma of others through stories, images, interactions, or by actually witnessing it happen. Individuals who experience secondary trauma are often extremely empathic. They have a strong sense of compassion that leads them to emotionally connect with and feel what others feel, whether pain, fear, or distress. They feel for others and sometimes this can affect them deeply.

Each type of trauma has a huge impact on how a person lives their life. And the process of healing and recovery varies depending on the severity of the trauma. Learning to recognize trauma is vital to providing appropriate care. You must also become knowledgeable about the types of trauma that accompany loss of a baby or pregnancy, such as acute trauma, grief and bereavement, complex grief, reproductive trauma, and social and cultural trauma.

- *Acute trauma*: This happens when a loss occurs unexpectedly, such as neonatal death, miscarriage, or stillbirth. Those who experience acute trauma manifest symptoms of acute stress and even PTSD (post-traumatic stress disorder) because of the shock and helplessness related to the occurrence.

- *Grief and bereavement*: The loss of a baby or pregnancy brings with it many different emotions and processes such as denial, anger, bargaining, depression, and acceptance (see Chapter 10 for more on grief and bereavement).

- *Complex grief*: This differs from grief and bereavement because it is accompanied by intense, prolonged, or complicating factors, such as unresolved trauma, strained relationships, and previous losses. In other words, there are many layers of other complex issues at hand, not just the loss of a baby or pregnancy. For instance, a woman who has a history of sexual abuse and physical assault may experience even greater and more intense grief when she loses a child during pregnancy or after. Why? There may be lack of healing, and facing loss may add to her past experiences and trauma. Thus, there are layers and layers of trauma all connected and relating to her body.

- *Reproductive trauma*: This is experienced by women who have a history of pregnancy losses or infertility issues. This type of trauma involves feelings of guilt, failure, and frustration. Women who experience this type of trauma are those that may be undergoing fertility treatments or those with a history of multiple miscarriages.

- *Social and cultural trauma*: This can occur when a woman feels like she has not met societal expectations or may feel like she is not living up to cultural beliefs. A stigma around pregnancy loss can contribute to additional layers of trauma. Thus, women experiencing social and cultural trauma may isolate themselves and feel judged and unsupported by those around them. It only magnifies their grief and trauma surrounding the loss of a child or pregnancy.

BIRTH WORKERS AND TRAUMA

Note that secondary trauma is not only reserved for those experiencing the loss. You will come to learn that attending births for any length of time will present many opportunities for secondary trauma to occur. It's important to have a level of self-awareness about the environment that you are walking into with your client, whether it be a hospital, birth center, or home space, and about the triggers that may be present there. Connecting with your clients and doing your due diligence on their background, history, and comfort level in their relationships will be key to helping you navigate these spaces. But most importantly: you must assess yourself.

When it comes to your personal triggers, it's important to do your best to show up as an objective supportive advocate for your clients. If we're not careful about our previous experiences with other clients, our personal experiences and outcomes, we'll skew our view and/or heighten our emotions in ways that may not best serve our clients. When it comes to forming relationships with our clients we must not stick to biases. We must detach from our experiences to broaden our perspective on any given situation. The more room we provide to accept others and learn from them, the more effective we can become.

Birth work means that you must immerse yourself in inner work. Again, processing and healing from trauma is not something that happens quickly. Being aware of our traumas and triggers is crucial. Awareness of what causes us to feel or respond in a certain way, helps us have agency, especially in tough situations.

One thing that is helpful is to conduct a self-assessment before meeting with your clients. Self-reflect and check your emotions. If you feel anxious or stressed in any way, immediately do something to release those emotions and tensions; that way you can show up with a clear mind open to help your clients. Engage in quick journaling sessions at the start of your day. It helps with revealing any thoughts that are causing stress or feelings of worry. Use the journaling process as your filter. How so? Let it all out on the page, negative and positive thoughts, and emotions. That way, when you do meet with your client, you are refreshed and ready to help them. So, don't forget to unpack and unload yourself, your thoughts, opinions, and any feelings that may disrupt your ability to provide optimal care.

Midwives, doulas, or anyone delivering a baby can experience secondary trauma because they are being exposed to traumatic events or outcomes. How do you know if you have been affected by secondary trauma? Let's explore the following factors.

- *Chronic stress*: As a birth worker, you will learn that the work is demanding on many levels. The nature of birth work involves high-pressure moments. This profession can contribute to chronic stress, and unaddressed chronic stress can lead to emotional burnout and exhaustion—resulting in secondary trauma.

- *Exposure to traumatic births*: Every birth is different, and, as a birth worker, you will witness beautiful moments just as much as complicated or traumatic births. Some examples of traumatic birth experiences are stillbirth, emergency cesarean sections, maternal complications, and fetal distress. You increase your chances of secondary trauma through repeated exposure to such events.

- *Emotional connections*: Birth workers form strong bonds with the mothers and their families, which means that our level of empathy is at one hundred percent. It makes birth workers the main source of support, making them even more vulnerable to internalizing emotional distress or that of their clients. Though something may affect you, you must be strong for the family or clients you are supporting. Internalizing emotions is never healthy, especially when prolonged, leading to secondary trauma.

- *Personal history*: There can also be a case where you have a history of trauma or loss, and when you witness and experience a traumatic birth, it may trigger you—thus compounding the trauma you experienced.

As mentioned before, prioritizing self-care and establishing healthy boundaries is crucial. You need to unpack, unload, heal, and seek support for your own mental health and well-being. The birth work profession is unpredictable, and you must be ready for anything. You need to know how to respond to even the worst of scenarios.

What will you do if you have the misfortune of having to navigate a loss with your client? I'm sure you've thought of how you would support the family through that difficult time, but have you considered how you yourself will navigate the grief you may feel or the trauma it may bring up?

Fortifying your heart and soul ahead of time is one of the greatest gifts you can give yourself and your clients. There is no way to prepare you for the sadness and despair that may arise in you as you hold space for others. Even when you have prepared and taken the training and courses that inform you on navigating pregnancy loss best, there's nothing like the moment when it becomes relevant. Though you have the theory and knowledge, nothing tops the actual experience of being there with your client facing a tough reality. Nothing prepares you for the waves of emotions you will encounter. However, you can learn as much as you can. The more knowledge, the more tools you have. And things will play out better for you and your client.

Showing up in the community as an emotional, spiritual, and phys-ical liaison can take its toll over time. It's so important that you build in time to rest, reset, and fill your own cup so that you can serve from your overflow. That can look different depending on your practice and what stage of life you're in. For some, it may look like taking a year off from birth work. For others, it may look like pivoting your services from in-person birth support to postpartum care. Whatever your needs are, ensure you keep your mental, emotional, and spiritual well-being at the forefront.

CHAPTER 9

Epigenetics in Pregnancy and Childbirth

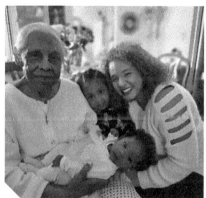
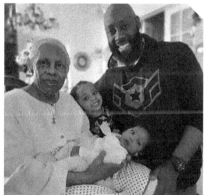

WHAT IS EPIGENETICS?

Epigenetics is the study of the impact of behaviors and environmental factors on inherited DNA expression. For example, if your grandfather had a certain type of behavior and you notice that your son exhibits the same behavior, it suggests that this trait was inherited through his genome, allowing him to express that habit from birth. Similarly, changes in behavior and modifications can be passed down through genetics when a traumatic event occurs. For instance, during the times of slavery in the United States, if a child displayed strength, intelligence, or any particular talent, they would often be chosen and sold away from their family. This practice had long-lasting effects, as discussed by Dr. Joy DeGruy in her book *Post Traumatic Slave Syndrome*. One of these effects is observed when Black mothers and children are in the presence of White families. The White mother may overemphasize the abilities of her child, causing an impulse in Black mothers to downplay their own child's talents and abilities in order to protect them. Although this impulse is no longer necessary for survival, it is still influenced by the imprints on our DNA from that time, which is known as epigenetics.

Epigenetics, in contrast to genetics, focuses on modifications of behavior that are passed down based on traumatic experiences. For example, research has shown that certain habits and behaviors developed by Jewish people during the Holocaust were still present in their descendants three generations later, even though these later generations had no direct exposure to the original traumatic events.[1] Similar studies have been conducted with mice, where they were conditioned to associate a specific smell, like peppermint, with a shock. Subsequent generations of mice still exhibited a physical reaction when exposed to the scent, even though they were not actually being shocked.[2] This demonstrates that epigenetics involves a modification of response and behavior based on traumatic events.

When considering the topic of pregnancy and childbirth, it is important to acknowledge the real challenges and present dangers faced by mothers. Additionally, we must also recognize the historical traumas experienced by mothers who had their babies forcibly taken from them or were victims of rape during conception. The pain and trauma endured during childbirth, as well as the conditions in which it occurred, can have a lasting impact. Depending on our family or generational history, our bodies may have a visceral response to something that happened to our ancestors, even if we find ourselves in a similar situation many years later.

Giving birth is a fundamental aspect of human existence, and it is crucial for us to understand the stories of our ancestors, acknowledge their traumas and pains, and actively work toward rewriting our genetic encoding. Just as generational traumas can be passed down in an epigenetic format, there are also generational blessings that can manifest in similar ways. This is why we observe certain patterns and behaviors within families. When it comes to birth work and supporting individuals dealing with collective and personal trauma, it is essential to recognize that what we see on the surface may be rooted in much deeper experiences.

Epigenetic modifications have the potential to be inherited. There are several factors that can influence these modifications. Environmental factors, such as habits, diet, and emotional well-being, play a significant role. When I mention environment, it encompasses how a person is raised, which brings us to the ongoing debate of nature versus nurture. In my opinion, it is a combination of both. This conversation never reaches a definitive conclusion, but I firmly believe that both nature and nurture contribute to epigenetic modifications.

For example, people often attribute certain health conditions like high blood pressure to their family history. However, it is crucial to consider the shared habits and dietary choices within the family. If everyone in your family consumes unhealthy foods and leads a sedentary lifestyle, it is not solely a genetic predisposition but also a result of learned behaviors. It is important to recognize that these factors can be changed by altering one's habits and lifestyle choices.

Additionally, certain traumatic events, not necessarily limited to physical trauma like a car accident, can trigger changes in gene expression. Emotional traumas, such as heartbreak, can also have an impact on DNA. Hormonal factors can also play a role, particularly in girls. If a girl comes from a family with a history of mental illness, she may not exhibit any signs of it until she reaches puberty and begins to experience hormonal changes. These expressions of mental illness or other traits may become more apparent during adolescence or early adulthood.

Epigenetic modifications can be influenced by other environmental factors. For instance, growing up in a suburban area where there is minimal exposure to law enforcement may result in a lack of fear or understanding of the police. However, if one day you find yourself in an environment surrounded by racist individuals, including a police officer, you may experience a physical and visceral reaction due to the sudden exposure to a different environment. This reaction is not based solely on personal experiences but can be influenced by the environment you find yourself in. It is rooted in something deeply ingrained within oneself, which I would describe as an epigenetic response. People may have fears or avoid certain things without any logical reasoning based on their personal experiences. However, these fears and avoidances can be attributed to the epigenetic history within their family, as habits of child rearing and parenting are passed down through generations. This can manifest in various aspects of life, affecting not only the individual but also their family and children.

EPIGENETICS AND ME

My introduction to the concept of epigenetics occurred during the early stages of my journey into motherhood. I attended a lecture at Morgan State University with Dr. Joy DeGruy, around the year 2007. She discussed her book *Post Traumatic Slave Syndrome*, and when she delved into the topic of epigenetics, it struck a chord with me. At that point in my motherhood journey, I followed every piece of advice given to me by my aunt, grandmother, and mother regarding my daughter. I believed that since they had raised me, I should do things exactly as they did. However, I began to question whether all of their methods truly resonated with me.

I didn't really think that it was actually healthy or that everything they said was necessarily right for my child. So when I heard that lecture, it opened up a brand new possibility for me to do things differently. I became curious about how my daughter was experiencing me. It was almost an out-of-body perspective, which I still have sometimes. If I'm caught up and having an angry response, and then I see my child have a visceral response, I'm like, "Oh my gosh!" I study them and wonder why they behaved that way. Many of my personal practices as a mother came into play based on my exposure to the understanding and concept of epigenetics in 2007 during that lecture.

Moving forward, when I became pregnant with my second daughter, I was in a very high-stress relationship, and I was hyper-aware of the potential traumatic effect it could have on my child. So I intentionally sat, meditated, breathed, and visualized a protective light around her and my belly to calm my nerves and regulate my nervous system. I didn't want her to be imprinted with that trauma. There were times when I could be coming out of an argument or feeling a certain way, but I knew the potential imprint it could have on my child, even before she was born. I had a level of awareness that made me think, "Oh my gosh, I need to do whatever I can about it." For me, at that point, it meant focusing on breathing and regulating my nervous system. Moving forward again to being pregnant with my son, it meant advocating for myself at a higher level. It meant protecting myself and setting boundaries.

In terms of interacting with the medical and healthcare system, I had an amazing OB for my older two children, who happened to be a Black woman. So intentionally, I chose to have Black women assist me with all of my children. However, for my son, I decided to have a Black midwife because I wanted someone who would honor my more holistic perspectives and desires for my birth experience. It also meant being clearer and more vocal in advocating for myself. I noticed that my body tensed up when certain nurses walked into the room, some of whom were White. Some of them treated me as if I didn't matter, and even though they may not have been explicitly rude, I had a physical response to them. I realized that there was more to it than just the present moment, and I didn't want to feel that way. So, I started asserting myself and saying, "You don't have permission to touch me" if someone was being rough or disrespectful. I remember one nurse being confused and asking, "What do you mean?" And I replied, "You don't have permission to touch me." She wondered how she would be able to complete her tasks without assistance, but I was adamant that nobody had permission to touch my body. This led to a process of self-discovery and finding tools to minimize negative impact and protect myself from expressing harmful emotions that would negatively impact my baby (i.e., stress and anger).

It was a journey that required acknowledging and confronting trauma, rather than succumbing to hopelessness. One crucial aspect was recognizing and addressing weak points in one's DNA, which everyone has but in different forms. However, simply acknowledging these weaknesses is not enough; behavioral and environmental changes are necessary to achieve different outcomes. For instance, living in a polluted city, drinking water with lead in it, and consuming processed food while hoping to avoid cancer, which others in my family have had, is unrealistic. Changing the environment and behavior is essential for a different result.

EFFECTS ON BIRTH OUTCOMES

When it comes to being a birth worker, it is crucial not to make assumptions or generalize about a client's experiences based on their race, such as assuming that all Black individuals have the same experiences. They must have grown up in a gang-ridden area, or perhaps there are other factors at play. It is not appropriate to make assumptions based on someone's ethnicity, such as assuming that a Latino person has multiple generations living in their house or questioning their legal status. These cultural and social judgments should not be made without taking the time to get to know the person and their story. By connecting with clients and understanding their background, we can gain insight into certain aspects that may influence their experiences, including epigenetics. It is important to remember that no ethnic group is a monolith, and individuals within each group have diverse backgrounds, countries of origin, beliefs, and religious perspectives.

By genuinely connecting with people and learning about their unique experiences, we can better support them through any challenges they may face during their birth experience.

It is therefore possible to mitigate negative impacts. This can be achieved through awareness and acknowledgment, as well as making changes in behavior, environment, diet, and emotional, mental, and psychological health. Seeking support in these areas, such as through somatic therapy, can be beneficial for individuals, particularly those from diverse backgrounds. Many people of color have healing practices rooted in movement, which can contribute to reversing the effects of epigenetics. Additionally, strengthening one's spiritual practice, regardless of the specific religious affiliation, can play a key role in this process.

Understanding the effects of diet is also important, going beyond cultural foods and discovering what truly nourishes and supports one's body. Nutrition is not only linked to physical health but also mental and spiritual well-being. For instance, a pregnant woman with a family history of gestational diabetes can make proactive choices during pregnancy to reduce her likelihood of experiencing it. This includes making healthy lifestyle choices and engaging in regular exercise.

Furthermore, it is crucial to consider stress-management techniques and tools for achieving balance and homeostasis. Each person is unique, and by understanding their individual needs and preferences, we can support them in being their authentic selves rather than merely a product of external influences.

There are also specific epigenetic factors that contribute to disparities in birth outcomes within the Black community. One significant factor stems from the historical trauma experienced during chattel slavery in the United States. Enslaved Black women, including African women, were forcibly separated from their newborns shortly after birth. In some cases, this separation was indefinite, leading to profound grief and emotional distress. Adding to the trauma, these women were often tasked with nursing the babies of their masters instead of their own, resulting in a deeply unsettling experience.

Even if a mother was allowed to keep her own child, she was often required to prioritize breastfeeding the master's baby over her own, potentially leading to a low milk supply for her own child. This historical context has had a lasting impact on breastfeeding disparities and the attitudes surrounding it in the Black community. There has been a stigma and a disconnect associated with breastfeeding, perpetuated by societal views that considered it as lowly or associated with poverty. This cultural disruption and disconnection between mothers and their babies has persisted through generations.

It is essential to recognize that prior to slavery, indigenous peoples and families worldwide viewed breastfeeding as a natural and honorable practice. Breastfeeding was deeply valued and cherished. However, the institutionalized slavery experience disrupted this cultural norm, leading to a ripple effect that continues to be felt today. Elders in the community may still express negative views towards breastfeeding due to the visceral response it evokes, reminding them of the painful history of having their babies forcibly taken away and being made to nurse someone else's child.

This traumatic history has not only left an epigenetic impact but has also influenced oral traditions and the passing down of advice between generations. It is crucial to acknowledge and address this historical context when discussing breastfeeding rates among indigenous and Black communities. By understanding the deep-rooted trauma and working towards healing and empowerment, we can strive for more equitable birth outcomes inside the Black community.

While specific epigenetic markers or patterns associated with adverse birth outcomes in Black individuals may vary, there are several contributing factors that have been identified. Poverty and lack of access to resources are significant factors that can lead to low birth weight, preterm birth, and stillbirth in the Black community. Similarly, indigenous communities also face challenges related to limited access to resources.

Food deserts, where there is a lack of grocery stores and reliance on processed foods, contribute to adverse birth outcomes. Additionally, inadequate access to comprehensive prenatal, pregnancy, and post-partum care can also impact birth outcomes. Lack of good jobs with benefits and transportation further exacerbate these challenges.

It is important to note that these contributing factors affect communities of color, particularly those in lower socioeconomic classes, more significantly. Research suggests that regardless of a Black person's economic standing, they may still face systemic issues and mistreatment in the healthcare system.[3, 4] While poor White women may also experience mistreatment, middle-class or upper-class White women are more likely to be treated with respect and given priority. Limited research is available on the different classes of Latina and Asian women, but it has been observed that indigenous and Black women, regardless of economic standing, tend to face poorer treatment.

Overall, addressing these systemic issues and disparities in access to resources and healthcare is crucial in improving birth outcomes in the Black community and other communities of color.

Epigenetic modifications can be used as biomarkers to predict or monitor the risk of certain birth complications in both poor White Caucasian women and Black women, as well as individuals from any other racial or ethnic background. The biomedical industry has made advancements in developing tests that can analyze specific markers in blood and DNA to provide information about predisposition to conditions like pre-eclampsia or preterm birth.

It is crucial to recognize the importance of such biomarkers in personalized healthcare. For example, the experience of my sister, who faced preterm birth with both of her pregnancies, highlights the need for healthcare providers to take into account an individual's history and potential genetic markers. Unfortunately, in my sister's case, the healthcare provider dismissed her concerns without conducting further investigations or considering her specific circumstances.

In addition to genetic markers, it is also important to consider physical conditions and other factors that may contribute to birth complications. Birth workers and healthcare providers should prioritize getting to know their clients on an individual level, understanding their unique histories, challenges, and potential risk factors. This personalized approach can help guide the development of a tailored care plan for each individual, taking into account their specific needs and potential risks based on epigenetic markers and other factors.

Intergenerational epigenetic inheritance plays a significant role in perpetuating disparities and birth outcomes in the Black community. When we fail to acknowledge the intergenerational impact and the history of systemic inequalities, we allow these disparities to persist. However, the current moment presents an opportunity for change.

By acknowledging and understanding our personal and collective histories, we can actively work toward breaking the cycle of intergenerational patterns. This requires a personal and collective effort to address the challenges and issues that have been passed down to us. The greatest impact will occur on a personal level, as individuals take the initiative to make changes in their own lives and challenge generational patterns.

Empowering individuals to be brave, courageous, and willing to confront the past is crucial. By doing so, they can create a different narrative and have the birth experiences they desire. It is inspiring to witness clients who become the first in their family to make positive changes and break generational patterns. For example, I recall supporting a young lady who had experienced self-harm and grew up in an unloving home. This individual's journey to change the narrative and have a different birth experience was a powerful example of personal responsibility and the potential for transformation.

To say that negative epigenetic expressions are irreversible, leaves little room for hope; it requires intentionality and doing the work to express different genes. Making different choices and placing yourself in different environments can cause different genetic expressions. It's like a repair or recalibration process.

As for epigenetic therapies that could potentially improve birth outcomes in marginalized communities, there aren't any available yet. It's an area that is currently being studied. However, personally, I believe that we don't have to wait for science. Indigenous practices that have been around for centuries, such as somatic healing, movement, dancing, crying, and releasing trauma from the body can all be beneficial. Surrounding oneself with community, love, and support can regulate the nervous system. When our nervous system is out of balance, it can lead to various health issues.

Community, movement, singing, and eating together are simple solutions that can have a profound impact. Cooking with nourishing herbs and feeding the body on a cellular level is important. These practices have been preserved in cultures that also celebrate and provide support during the postpartum period. For example, I met a Somalian woman during an accelerated program, and she mentioned that in her culture, there is no word for postpartum depression. It is expected that when someone in their community has a baby, the young women in the community go in rotation to support her. She recalled a time her mother sent her and her sister to provide support without any questions asked. The older women in the community teach them what to do. In such a culture, where women automatically support the new mother by cooking, massaging her feet, bathing her, and ensuring her well-being, there is no need for a term like postpartum depression. This is because the person has access to food, community, laughter, and love. When these elements are present, certain genetic expressions have a decreased opportunity to manifest. Unfortunately, Black and Brown communities in the United States and abroad have not had much access to these elements.

Overall, addressing intergenerational epigenetic inheritance requires a deep understanding of personal stories, histories, and the willingness to challenge and change the patterns that have been passed down. It is through individual empowerment and collective efforts that we can work towards improving birth outcomes and reducing disparities within the Black community.

EPIGENETICS RESEARCH

I believe that the scientific and research community is slowly starting to delve deeper into the issue of addressing racial disparities in maternal and infant health. With this acknowledgement comes accountability. Once we begin to explore the correlation between poor maternal and infant outcomes and epigenetic expression, it will become evident that there is a significant problem. It will be a challenging task to uncover how many people have been mistreated, how many unnecessary infant deaths have occurred, and how much stress has been embedded in the medical system. There is a level of accountability that comes with this realization. We are responsible for the systems we create, how we treat people, and how we interact with them on both personal and systemic levels. As we deepen our understanding of epigenetics and involve diverse voices and perspectives, it will become clear that we need to treat expectant mothers better, provide them with support, and minimize their stress levels. It's not just about the mothers; the babies are also being impacted.

What ethical considerations should be taken into account when conducting epigenetics research related to birth in the Black community or marginalized communities? One crucial consideration is personal bias. Researchers must make a concerted effort to check their biases and ensure that the research team is diverse, not just racially but also experientially. Currently, research is predominantly conducted within a White arena, which means that there is a lack of accurate insights and information. This highlights the importance of having a diverse research team in any country, university, or subject, particularly when it comes to maternal and infant health.

How do social determinants of health, such as racism and socioeconomic status, influence genetic modifications related to birth outcomes? It's like compound interest. When you are poor and belong to a marginalized community, such as being Black, Brown, a person of color, or an immigrant in this country, each of these conditions alone puts you at risk for poor health outcomes. When you have two or more of these factors, such as being poor, Black, and a woman, the risks multiply. You are more likely to experience pre-eclampsia, fear of stillbirth, medical coercion, dismissiveness, obstetrical violence, pediatric violence, and cultural violence in the form of the involvement of child protection services. There are various ways in which individuals are bullied, stressed, and pushed into a state of fight or flight, leading to constantly elevated cortisol levels and perpetual stress. In a non-pregnant body, this is enough to be life-threatening, but in a pregnant body, it can be fatal for both the mother and the baby. This is exactly what we are witnessing in minority communities. It is important to note that communities of color are actually the global majority, but due to systemic racism and other oppressive practices, we are seeing mothers and babies lose their lives.

NOTES

1   Dashorst, P., Mooren, T.M., Kleber, R.J., de Jong, P.J., and Huntjens, R.J.C. (2019) "Intergenerational consequences of the Holocaust on offspring mental health: A systematic review of associated factors and mechanisms." *European Journal of Psychotraumatology* 10, 1, 1654065. doi:10.1080/20008198.2019.1654065

2   Dias, B.G. and Ressler, K.J. (2014) "Parental olfactory experience influences behavior and neural structure in subsequent generations." *Nature Neuroscience* 17, 1, 89–96. doi:10.1038/nn.3594

3   Macias-Konstantopoulos, W.L., Collins, K.A., Diaz, R., Duber, H.C., *et al.* (2023) "Race, healthcare, and health disparities: A critical review and recommendations for advancing health equity." *Western Journal of Emergency Medicine* 24, 5, 906–918.

4   Jackson, P.B. and Cummings, J. (2011) "Health Disparities and the Black Middle Class: Overview, Empirical Findings, and Research Agenda." In B.A. Pescosolido, J.K. Martin, J.D. McLeod, and A. Rogers (eds) *Handbook of the Sociology of Health, Illness, and Healing* (pp.383–410). New York, NY: Springer.

CHAPTER 10

Understanding Grief

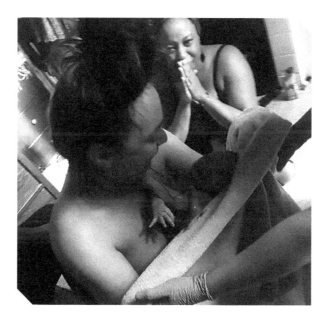

Grief and trauma are overwhelming responses to loss. It's something that everyone will endure at some point in their life. Birth work is no different. Over the last few years, it seems as though we've all dealt with some level of grief or trauma. We've navigated a pandemic, experienced illness, and faced losing loved ones. It is even possible to grieve who we once were.

Many of us are currently living in a state and cycle of continuous grief, grieving old versions of ourselves. It's because of this reality concerning grief that it is more important than ever to take care of our mind. We must equip ourselves with healthy tools to navigate, maintain, heal, and grow through each transition and season in our lives to live with greater peace amid grief and trauma. Though we cannot control what happens to us or those we care about, we can control how we respond to the struggles that arise.

THE BIRTHING EXPERIENCE

As we all know, the process of giving birth to a child is unpredictable. In the modern world, many outcomes are possible every time someone goes into labor. As a birth worker, you are responsible for holding space for your clients and their families. It's important to show up with a clean slate, a clear heart, and a clear mind, if only for a moment. Each family comes to the table with a set of experiences, fears, and concerns that may show up in ways you could never predict! Only adding more unpredictability to the entire birth experience.

For instance, if a family has experienced the loss of a child during a past pregnancy, there will be subtle or overt fears throughout the pregnancy. A woman or family that has experienced loss will face different struggles than those who have not. As a birth worker, you are their support system. You must help them navigate all fears and challenges concerning birthing their child early on in the pregnancy.

However, not all feelings and emotional challenges concerning the loss of a child in a past pregnancy or pregnancies can be processed within the span of nine to ten months. In situations like this, you will find that emotional and spiritual support make their way to the forefront. You must hold a space for your clients, which means that you will provide them with the emotional support and freedom for them to ask questions. In turn, you must approach them carefully, probing gently to attain as much information as you can to support them according to their needs. Supporting your clients in the best way possible becomes a dance that you do with each family according to what they need most, whether information, guidance, someone who can listen to them, empathy, understanding, or all the above.

Since every woman and their family grieve differently, every client and their birth experience will differ. So, you must become knowledgeable on this topic of grief. You must know how people cope and how they manage strong waves of emotions and thoughts that come with it.

THE STAGES OF GRIEF

It is important to familiarize yourself with the basic understanding of grief and trauma. In doing so, you will show up at your best and support the families you serve at the highest level. As stated in previous chapters, personal development is a key part of capacity building as a birth worker. Your willingness and openness to understand, learn, and study concepts and perspectives that broaden your personal worldview will ultimately make you a greater resource for the families you serve. The more you know, the more of an asset you will be throughout the birthing experience, especially during labor.

There are five stages of grief: Denial, Anger, Bargaining, Depression, and Acceptance. The concept of five stages of grief was originally introduced by a psychiatrist named Elisabeth Kübler-Ross in 1969. Although all five stages are not universally experienced in the same way by every woman and their family, there can be a combination of these stages in any woman experiencing grief over the loss of someone they love, especially when it relates to a child.

First stage: Denial

In the first stage, for a woman who has faced the loss of a child it is natural for her to reject the idea that the loss is true and to accept that it actually took place. The reality is that women process trauma and grief in many ways. Because a woman might be in denial, it may lead her to avoid conversations with others or reminders of the truth, thus causing her to isolate herself. Denial is a defense mechanism that provides emotional protection from the shock of the loss. Think of it like a temporary buffer that minimizes the intensity of the pain.

Second stage: Anger

The next stage of the grief process is the intense feeling of anger. As soon as a woman experiences the numbness of denial beginning to wear off, it is replaced with feelings of anger. Frustration kicks in, leading a woman to direct her anger towards themselves, others, their spouse, or the child they lost. We must note that with the loss of a child, the father will go through these stages of grief as well, and cannot be ignored. Anger is a natural response to a woman's helplessness in such an unfair situation. Loss of an unborn child is not something anyone expects, nor is it a wound that can be healed quickly. It's a delicate matter.

Third stage: Bargaining

During this stage of the grief process, women and even their spouses may make deals. What does this mean? They might begin to pray or promise to change their behavior if only the child they lost could come back. The underlying motivator behind the bargaining is the need to regain control of the situation or attempt to change the outcome. Bargaining is a defense mechanism against feelings of helplessness.

For instance, a woman or her spouse may seek to negotiate within themselves, with others around them, with fate, the universe, or a higher power to change their circumstances. This type of mental state consists of high levels of rumination over the details of the loss. A woman and even her spouse may spend much time seeking to understand why the loss of their child happened.

The bargaining stage is a season in which a woman and their partner are desperately trying to make sense of the loss and revisit the past to see what or where they went wrong. They may even experience guilt, manifesting in how they try to be better by helping others, volunteering, and even making donations to deal with the pain.

Fourth stage: Depression

In this stage of grief, there are overwhelming feelings of sadness because the full weight of the loss settles. Many women have described their depression as a deep sorrow and anguish. It's an indescribable pain that can even manifest in the form of physical pain. In this stage, a woman, and even her partner, must seek professional help because there is such a thing as clinical depression and grief over the loss of a loved one.

Fifth stage: Acceptance

The final stage is acceptance. It's when a grieving mother and the father come to terms with the loss of their child. When a mother accepts the loss of her baby or unborn child it does not mean that she has stopped grieving and hurting. It means that they have come to terms with their reality. Experts say that grief can last a lifetime after a major loss. However, coping with the loss only becomes easier with time. It's important to note that grief can manifest in the form of waves, where a mother is triggered by reminders of the loss long after she has accepted it. These triggers can set a woman off to cross over into any of the other four stages of grief.

MEN AND GRIEF

Men and how they grieve are often overlooked when dealing with the loss of a past pregnancy or child. One reason for this oversight can be the prevailing societal expectations and stereotypes around masculinity. Men are often expected to be stoic, strong, and less emotionally expressive. This societal belief places unnecessary pressure on men and may discourage them from openly discussing their emotions amid grief. It may even deter them from seeking support, leading them to suffer silently. Sadly, many men feel the need to be strong for their wives or partners, leading them to suppress their emotions. Consequently, their grief can go unnoticed or misunderstood by others, including their partners, family, and friends, who may assume that they are handling the loss well when, in reality, they are struggling.

It's vital that, as a birth worker, you do not overlook a woman's partner, because men do grieve. The healing process is not linear or unbending. It is a nuanced and complicated process. Two grieving parents can sway in and out of stages of grief at different times while experiencing similar emotions along the way. In fact, not everyone goes through all the stages of grief. So, you need to know how to identify what stage someone is at in the grieving process. That way, you know how to respond.

HOW TO RESPOND ACCORDING TO THE STAGES OF GRIEF

If you have identified that a woman is in the denial stage for the loss of a past pregnancy, you must be patient. Gentle reassurance that you are there to support her in any way you can is helpful. Avoid pressuring her to confront her feelings if she is not ready. Encourage open communication and offer information and support resources when she is ready.

If you can tell that the woman you are treating is in the anger stage and expressing anger toward the loss, it's up to you to validate her emotions. Let her know it is okay to feel angry and reinforce that her emotions are natural. Be nonjudgmental and become an empathic listener. Offer her and her spouse a safe space to vent their frustrations and ask if they would like suggestions for healthy ways to cope with anger. Healthy ways to cope with anger are exercise, journaling, prayer, coloring, painting, and taking a creative class of some sort.

If the woman in your care is in the bargaining stage of grief, then you know that she and even her partner are most likely focused on thoughts of "what could have been done differently?" Become a listening ear and validate her feelings. Encourage her to talk about her regrets. If you notice she is receptive, then help her explore the idea that grief does not follow any set of rules. Her experience is unique to her and her journey.

If you notice that the woman and her spouse are facing signs of deep sorrow and depression and seem isolated from others, create a strong support system for them. Provide resources for grief counseling or therapy. Encourage them to seek professional help if you notice that their depression becomes persistent and overwhelming.

And lastly, if you have identified that the woman in your care, and even their partner, are in the acceptance stage of the grief process, then celebrate that progress. Offer continued support and even encourage her to find ways to honor the loss of their child.

THE POWER OF CREATIVE OUTLETS

Let's face it: there is only so much you can do despite the amount of information you may have. You can be a listening ear and someone who validates emotions, but most of the work toward healing must be done by the person enduring the grieving process. Therefore, one of the most powerful things you can do to help a woman and her partner is to encourage them to engage in creative outlets. Direct them toward the things that will help them heal.

Encourage your client to engage in creative processes, because creativity ignites self-expression. Therefore, it can provide a safe space for exploring complex feelings that may be difficult to express verbally. For instance, when someone is engaged in creating art, it allows them to externalize their inner struggles and find catharsis in the act of creation. When a person dives into a catharsis state, they can release pent-up emotions and find a sense of relief.

Relief leads to reduced stress in the midst of a stress-inducing situation. When people dive into creative processes, it leads to a state of flow where they become deeply immersed and focused on the activity that they are doing. This can temporarily alleviate some of the stress they feel and produce a sense of calm and relaxation, especially for the ruminating mind. Creativity can help provide rest for the aching heart.

Creative activities can also foster a sense of agency as a woman and her partner are trying to regain control of their emotions. Encourage creative outlets because they can serve as powerful tools for healing and personal growth, especially after losing a child. In fact, if a woman were to partake in an art or painting class, this can help her foster social connection, and this is extremely helpful if the woman and her partner have been isolating themselves from others. Group activities like art therapy or anything that brings people together provide a sense of community.

Research has suggested that creative expression can contribute to psychological healing and resilience.[1, 2] It can help individuals make sense of their experiences, find meaning in adversity, and move forward with a sense of purpose and strength. Neuroscientific studies have shown that engaging in creative activities can stimulate various regions of the brain associated with emotion regulation and problem-solving, leading to improved emotional well-being.[3, 4, 5]

This information is important for you to know as a birth worker because the more knowledge you have of what helps a person navigate grief in a healthier manner, the more of an asset you become to the woman and her family. You become a key point of contact and support.

Overall, become an active listener and never forget to care for yourself as a birth worker. Helping someone or multiple people through grief can be emotionally challenging. It can lead you to an emotionally charged mental state. Care for yourself and make sure that you process your own feelings and reactions to the situation at hand.

NOTES

1   Xu, Y., Shao, J., Zeng, W., Wu, X., *et al.* (2021) "Depression and creativity during COVID-19: Psychological resilience as a mediator and deliberate rumination as a moderator." *Frontiers in Psychology* 12, 665961.

2   Davis, J. (2020, June 16) "How creativity builds resilience in times of crisis." *Psychology Today*. www.psychologytoday.com/us/blog/tracking-wonder/202006/how-creativity-builds-resilience-in-times-crisis

3   Khalil, R., Godde, B., and Karim, A.A. (2019) "The link between creativity, cognition, and creative drives and underlying neural mechanisms." *Frontiers in Neural Circuits* 13, 18.

4   Park, S.H., Kim, K.K., and Hahm, J. (2016) "Neuro-scientific studies of creativity." *Dementia and Neurocognitive Disorders* 15, 4, 110–114.

5   Zhou, K. (2018) "What cognitive neuroscience tells us about creativity education: A literature review." *Global Education* 5, 1, 20–34.

CHAPTER 11

❖◇◇◇◇◇◇◇◇◇◇◇◇◇◇◇◇◇❖

Becoming

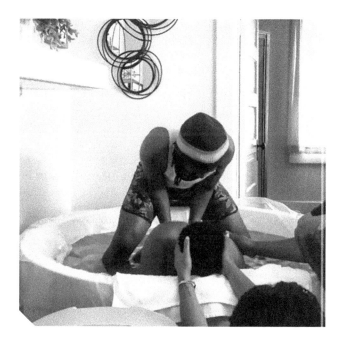

FINDING MY CALLING

I did not start my journey as a birth worker because I was interested in that kind of work. Instead, it was a feeling that evolved from the moment I started supporting my friend who got pregnant straight out of high school. She had a very tumultuous pregnancy and birth, exacerbated by interesting interactions with her family. I distinctly remember the moment when we were all at the bottom of the steps in her parents' house, and someone approached her. They were checking on her and asking about the baby, putting their hand on her stomach, saying, "How is MY such and such?"

My friend responded, "Can you not touch my stomach?" That person got offended. It was an appalling exchange. My friend had the right to her body and to voice when she felt uncomfortable, yet she was so easily dismissed. I was the outsider looking in on this situation, sitting in the front row of this predicament during this vulnerable season of her life. I remember the frustration on her face masked as irritation.

After, I would ask her things like, "Do you want me to take you to your doctor's appointments? Do you want me to do your nails? Do you want me to get you out of here, even if it's just to go to the store?" I started checking in on her consistently throughout her pregnancy, and it was natural because we were friends. When she went into labor, we were all at the hospital with her, and, by all, I mean all of her immediate family members and myself. She was the first of our friend group to get pregnant, so none of us knew what to expect.

We were young, I was 19 and she was 18. There was a point in her labor when I started to pray because we all got kicked out of the birthing room. They were speaking about prepping her for an emergency c-section. During her stay she was administered Pitocin, among other medications. I remember being afraid for my friend because I thought she would undergo surgery, but things turned around. As a final measure, the doctor gave her an episiotomy, and the baby was born.

Once she was in the postpartum room, things were tense. They had given her so many drugs she could barely hold her baby. Then, an argument with the child's father exploded. I remember the flurry of insults, screaming, and all-around violence that took place while in that room with the baby. And again, I'm standing there, a third party, witnessing this whole situation.

My friend cried and said, "I can't even hold my baby. I want to breastfeed my baby. That's the only thing that I wanted out of this whole thing. I feel like none of this has happened the way that I wanted it to go." She just cried. I never forgot this. I even offered to spend the night with her. There were so many factors in this experience that impacted me greatly.

I remember walking away from that situation with many thoughts, for many different reasons. I walked away believing that birth was beautiful, marvelous, and wonderful, but only in the absence of certain barriers. Witnessing birth has been amazing every time, but witnessing trauma happening in that situation sparked something in me. I knew I didn't want others to experience that level of trauma, especially not during such a fragile time.

From that birth forward, I became an advocate for the girls and the women in my life and family. I attended every birth in some capacity from that point on when someone in my circle became pregnant. Life would have it that I was the next one to get pregnant. Because of what I'd witnessed, I opted for a supportive birth team and employed natural and holistic practices.

Pregnancies, for me, became an opportunity to walk in my calling. I believe I was called for such a profession. It tugged at my heart throughout the years until it came to fruition. And now, I strive to give the best of myself through continuous radical growth and learning. One of the most profound findings I've had while I've been on my journey as a birth worker is the need to understand the human psyche. To understand the human mind is relevant to the work we do daily. As we deal with women and families, we get the chance to experience and understand what makes us different and unique; this helps develop compassion. Not to mention that as we expand as birth workers we make room to empathize with the pain and processes of others. This work stretches you in ways you may not have thought possible. I believe it's because, as a birth worker, you are involved and play an important, supportive role during such a sacred event in someone's life—the birth of a child, a new life that comes to this world.

As a result, we come to appreciate and welcome the differences that exist from person to person, family to family. What we do with those differences determines whether we build doors or barriers. We have a choice to make with every interaction we have. We can build doors that will allow open communication or barriers that may block the flow of comfort-filled connections.

I've come to understand that, though everyone we may encounter is different in this field, we all have three things in common. *Each of us seeks support, security, and comfort.* The knowledge of this commonality can help us move beyond our personal perspectives and biases and make room for others. And to make room for others, we must shift toward becoming inclusive and culturally sensitive to each family we serve.

CULTURAL SENSITIVITY AND INCLUSION

What does it mean to be culturally sensitive and inclusive? We all have different backgrounds, cultures, and upbringings, ultimately shaping our worldview and who we are. To serve our clients best, we must immerse ourselves in learning about who they are, and we can do so through inquisitive conversations and light probing. We must become more interested in learning about who they are than having them learn about us.

One way we can ensure that our services are culturally sensitive and inclusive is by connecting authentically with the individual family we're serving. We must do our best not to assume perspectives based on race or background, and for me, it's been helpful. If we purpose to stay away from assumptions and instead listen with an open mind, we'd be surprised at what we find. I've had the honor of serving a lot of intercultural families, such as Latino and Asian. I've had that mix a couple of times—Asian, Latino, African American, White American, Black Caribbean, and Black American, and so on.

You can't ever really tell just by the looks of people what cultural sensitivity or inclusion feels like to them. One of the best ways to approach this aspect of our work is in consultations and during our prenatal appointments. Leading with a deep dive into who they are and their family dynamics growing up can reveal valuable insights. You can try to discover their religious or non-religious practices and what has impacted them as a couple and as individuals. Getting to know your clients on such levels can inform you on how you will need to show up for them.

There is no cookie-cutter way that we show up for our clients. Different families may experience us in different ways. Depending on their needs, some people want us to be very involved and become close, like a family member. Other people like us to be less connected and to play a more distant role. Some people prefer interactions that mirror their experiences with medical professionals, less personal or intimate.

It's essential to get to know each couple, their background, and their preferences. It is crucial to ask questions about who they are and connect with them based on what they tell you about themselves. It's up to us to find out what they might need from us and their birth experience. In other words, we must become client-centered and extremely focused on getting to know them at deeper levels. It requires getting to know who they are and following your intuition. This process also requires observing how they respond to us in different environments and situations, and while discussing specific topics.

It is also important to understand the basic tenets of culturally responsive care. One must connect with the client, including becoming an attentive listener—being slow to speak and quick to listen. As we listen, we make space for people to tell us about themselves and share their stories. You can read between the lines and identify specific needs in their stories. People will let you know what solutions they need and what they are looking for, even when they are not describing the solution in a direct way. In addition, stories show us a person's individuality, perspectives, and beliefs.

In fact, the stories people share help us see certain patterns in behavior and coping mechanisms. As we identify personality traits and behavior patterns, we can identify weaknesses and strengths. But also, we can understand how people may feel about certain situations. It's psychological. People do not realize how much psychology goes into birth work.

Each woman and family provides you with information about who they are, and it's up to you to put those pieces together to make sense of the entire picture of who they are and what they need. It's like putting puzzle pieces together. It's also almost like being a detective. You must find what makes your clients tick, what is calming to them, and what types of situations may be threatening or trigger negative emotions that could lead to a negative experience.

Remarkably, people will tell you what they need if you listen closely to their narratives and how they communicate what has brought them pain or joy. It's vital to identify a person's needs instead of making assumptions. When you avoid assumptions, you create a more inclusive environment, interaction, and culturally sensitive space. The goal is to help your clients feel welcomed as they are, as their most authentic selves.

In each interaction with our clients, we must be sure to show up as ourselves. Don't try to bend or mold yourself to become like the cultures you serve, but give them the respect that you would like, which builds a foundation of mutual respect and communication between you and them. The more authentic we are, the more authentic they can be. People can tell when you are being genuine. Leading with a genuine attitude will help increase the chances of clients opening up to you, which is what you want.

If all else fails in conversation, there is one thing you can always count on. The following theme is consistent across cultures worldwide, and that one theme is food. No matter where you are from, you can always talk about food. We all need and enjoy food; inquiring about what specific cultural foods make us feel loved and comforted is a good starting point for any conversation. Conversations are psychological. You must build rapport and an avenue of communication by sparking connections based on commonalities, and if there's one thing we can all agree on, eating is enjoyable; but we love to talk about the foods we find most delightful too. Our faces light up when we talk about our favorite cuisine.

In most cases, you will never talk about food in a low-energy tone. On the contrary, people will give you all the details on recipes and restaurants they like to visit frequently. In fact, it's a good topic of conversation to build on and pursue other topics. It can bring up other topics of conversation like upbringing, childhood, and family relationships. The more we know about our clients, the better we can serve and support them.

It's also wise to find out what community looks like for them and some of their cultural taboos. Why community?, you might ask. Knowing what they consider to be a community can provide insight into the kind of support system they have in place, or if they lack support from family and friends. It also provides insight as to what they feel comfortable with. When people talk about their families, you can identify the dynamics, whether they have healthy, toxic, or average familial relationships or friendships.

For instance, if a woman says she doesn't talk to her family much and she only has her spouse or one good friend, these details tell me that this woman may be a private person and may prefer intimate settings. Therefore, their birth experience must be as intimate as possible. This information can also inform you that they may rely on you for sole support since they have a small support system.

When someone talks about their family, you can also determine beliefs and perspectives, helping you identify how to approach certain topics of conversation with sensitivity. For instance, if you have a woman and family who say that they don't believe in a higher power (God), yet you hold beliefs that contradict theirs, it helps you become aware of what you can say or must refrain from saying. In a scenario such as this one, you already know that sharing your personal beliefs about God is not something you should do because you must be sensitive to their beliefs. You are there to serve them, not persuade them to adopt your belief system.

The more you ask, the more information you will gather. A client's answers to your questions will only come from having genuine conversations and engaging with people from a place of authenticity. And it's an important part of the process. We gain information through conversations and observations—in a culturally sensitive and inclusive manner. In other words, we become skillful observers.

ADVOCATING FOR CLIENTS

There are always moments when we must advocate for our clients, but, in terms of what strategies we should employ in that regard, it's more about teaching and educating our clients on self-advocacy. Having honest and mindful conversations helps our clients recognize their challenges and weak spots. It also helps make them aware of their strengths, and we can assist with directing them to the right resources.

It is not about changing anyone. These mindful conversations help us determine what gaps we can fill and what needs must be met. I have found that during these conversations, you might want to introduce new concepts that are different from how this person has been living life. Although the goal is not to enter someone's life with the intention to change everything, we must introduce new concepts as new options that a person can choose to live more fully and peacefully, especially throughout a birth journey.

You don't want to go into someone's life, and they're five months pregnant, and have them do a whole lifestyle overhaul. That's not going to work; as a matter of fact, it may come across as intrusive. And we don't want people to feel invaded. What you want to do is come in and understand where they are. Assess that as accurately as possible, get the lay of the land and then see where the gaps are and how those gaps can be filled by you or other support members like their spouse, their partner, their friends, their parents, their community members, and their other loved ones. This process of advocating and helping your client make the right changes for their well-being and that of their unborn child will look different for every family.

One of the things that I've found useful time and time again is to pursue conversations and advice from a place of encouragement. By encouraging our clients, we help them to get in tune with themselves. We don't come in as an expert on their body and an expert on their needs. We come in as someone seeking to learn and understand what they already know and have experienced about themselves. It's a different thing to come as someone who wants to help in every way possible. It helps clients become vulnerable because they feel like their story, who they are, what they need, and what they feel, are valued. Making your client feel valued and seen is one of the most special things you can do for someone.

I would say decentering yourself as a doula and birth worker is key. Staying curious and asking directed questions and then really leaning into empowering those families, couples, and individuals into speaking up for themselves and what they need. Communication is really at the core when it comes to educating families on how to become advocates for themselves. We often don't consider how people are reared and how uncomfortable people might be with speaking up for themselves. And when you really get to talk, you know and understand that where we must focus our support is in the communication department. We must teach women, couples, and families to advocate for themselves and talk firmly without fear about their concerns and what they need. It is a whole self-development piece that many don't realize is essential to the birthing experience. The birthing journey is one where people do not consider how vulnerable they become because of the sensitive nature of labor.

Once a person or family learns how to advocate for themselves, they become empowered to communicate their feelings and needs more clearly and boldly. So, part of the self-development piece of helping clients is empowering their voice and sense of autonomy. In my practice, I have people practice within their relationships. Why? Because people will say things like: "I have a hard time with this thing or person. I have a hard time telling my children something. I have a hard time communicating with my husband."

When I hear what they are struggling with in their communication, that's when I lead them to practice their communication skills with those closest to them. That way, when they get to the hospital or the birth center or interact with different health professionals, they will have a decreased level of fear and be more comfortable communicating what they think or feel about something in the moment.

Give homework to your clients in an area where you feel they are most uncomfortable. It's important to work on strengthening their areas of insecurity and weakness. Make communication exercises a part of their daily practice. Make sure that each client asks themselves the following: Can you draw better boundaries with your mother-in-law, mother, sisters, children, husband, spouse, or partner?

Leading your clients to identify the root of their discomfort is a practice that will pay dividends when the waves of labor begin. Mindfulness is important. Ask them questions like: Where is that discomfort coming from physically? Do you feel it in your chest? Do you feel it in your gut? Do you feel your heart start racing? What's going on with your body? The answers to these questions can help us determine if they are having an anxious response to someone or something. It lets us know if people are pushing past boundaries or if they are doing too much. If the physical response is severe, we can determine whether we may need to seek additional mental health support to help the client navigate special circumstances.

Anxious or negative responses also indicate the need for physical movements, such as light exercise, dancing, or something enjoyable that will release endorphins. Consider leading your clients to think about the areas of their lives they have been neglecting. Probe and ask them to self-reflect on what makes them feel powerful, beautiful, and grounded. Lead them to think about the things that produce high confidence levels. Be sure to prompt them to revisit those things that make them feel alive and purposeful.

It's important to encourage them to continue or pick up those things they enjoy doing most. The things that bring the most joy and make them feel comfortable in their own skin. Motivate them to integrate those practices in small ways. If they love to dance, they can turn up the music and dance around the house and the kitchen. They can even take up a dance class with light moves, too. Once they have completed this homework, they can evaluate how they truly feel. It's these little simple solutions, and daily habitual practices that help them figure out what works and what areas need more work to get them to where they need to be—in a healthier emotional and mental state.

A part of this process of helping a client get to a better place is the practice of affirmations—phrases, verses, mantras, or sayings that evoke peace, calm, and focus when repeated; they are able to elicit feelings of calm and groundedness during moments of stress and discomfort, especially in labor. With affirmations, I lean on my client's preferences. There is also the matter of hypnobirthing programs. These programs look at focusing one's mind to decrease pain and enhance the likelihood of achieving the birth that is desired through visualization. The basis of these concepts is repetition.

The point of hypnobirthing is to tap into the subconscious mind. We often think we're making decisions from our conscious minds, but the reality is that our subconscious mind guides our actions. And so, if you can get certain information into your subconscious mind through repetition, that will guide your actions without you thinking about it. This is specifically a vital component of the birth experience: to train your mind to adopt certain thoughts that will enhance the birthing experience in a positive way through embedded subconscious thoughts.

One of the other tools and practices that has worked out amazingly among my clients who really took this practice seriously, is writing out notecards with their chosen Bible verses, affirmations, or goals. Clients should carve out five minutes out of their day to repeat those Bible verses, affirmations, and goals, then meditate on these things and take time for prayer.

When the moment of birth comes, and they have done the homework given them, there is a physical decrease in pain. They have had a boost in confidence and persistence to achieve what they set out to achieve. They have been able to practice cultivating a positive mindset through Bible verses, affirmations, and mindfulness exercises. They can go into their zone more easily since they have already been practicing. Interestingly, I can always tell who hasn't done their homework because things in the subconscious mind arise and begin to shatter their original plans for that birth moment.

Unless you have trained, trained, and retrained leading up to the birth, it's unfair to expect the most positive of outcomes. As doulas, we must help our clients with their communication and help them feel empowered to self-advocate. Believe it or not, mindfulness and affirmations impact birth outcomes and can support or interfere with what a client would like to experience. These are two major tools and practices that I use consistently. They can always be tweaked and curated to the specific family you are serving.

BEING A DOULA

This book is something I was inspired to write to help you explore the ins and outs of this profession and what you can expect. The publisher created this book's title based on an article I wrote for Healthline called "A Black Doula's Role in Improving Birth Outcomes." In that article, I talked about concrete things that Black women need in terms of support and birth, and when you think about the title of this book, *A Doula's Guide to Improving Maternal Health for BIPOC Woman*, it does not matter what race you are. If you are a Ukrainian or Ecuadorian doula, African American or Asian birth worker, we need you. None of it matters at the core—background, ethnicity, or race. We need you whole and ready to serve and support!

The point is to serve women and their families well. The point is to seek to understand the nuances and the uniqueness of their experiences. That is what will allow us as doulas to support them at a high level. That's what allows me, as a Black and indigenous woman, to serve women of all backgrounds. I have served Caucasian, Latina, Asian, African American, and Caribbean women, etc. well. And it's not because of my race. It's not because we share the same skin tone. It's not because we share the same or similar lived experiences. Nor is it because of the beautiful exchanges that we have shared throughout the birthing journey.

I do what I do and strive to serve each client well because of the principles that I talk about here in this book. I'm committed personally to radical growth and understanding of myself, which allows me to commit to a radical understanding of others. If we can understand where our client is emotionally or mentally, we can help them, educate them, and guide them. We can also have compassion and empathy for them to help them feel understood, heard, respected, and honored.

However, if we were to show up with an elevated ego as the expert on everything, we would tell our clients what they need based on our own assumptions without listening to them intently. It is different when we position ourselves, not as an expert but as an inquisitive ally who wants to support. What we want to create is something opposite to a doctor's visit—a visit with a physician who presumes to know exactly what you need without listening to you. That is not the kind of birth worker you are.

If a client wants to be seen by a doctor, then by all means that is what they should do. But if they want someone to love, support, and walk alongside them on their journey, they need someone with a more humane outlook on the birthing experience. A client seeking a natural, more humane experience for the birth of their baby needs someone in tune with their feelings. They need someone to be able to connect with them and communicate at a deeper level. Some clients desire to be connected to someone who understands every aspect of them pre-, during, and post-pregnancy. Someone who is invested in their emotional and mental health and well-being because all of those things are going to come into play at that pivotal moment of giving birth and bringing that baby earthside.

And so, for me, this book is a beacon of encouragement to help others become better, to serve better. It's a call to help women experience enriching moments through birthing. This book stands to empower doulas to know the impact they have on women and their families. It's an impact that can last a lifetime. There are no memories like the ones where you brought another life into this world. It's one of the most important experiences within a family unit. And if you can show up being your best, giving your best, it can make all the difference in someone's life and beyond.

One of the best ways to serve women and their families is to stay curious about people. I love people. I love people-watching everywhere I go. I may look at someone and wonder what makes this person tick, what makes them happy, what empowers them. Maintaining that curiosity makes space for your clients and influences how good a listener you are to those you serve. I further cultivate the need to want to know my clients, how their family dynamics work, and identify what is most important to them.

As a doula, I've become a lifelong learner, not only learning how to improve but also how to understand the minds of others, their responses, and the root of their reactions. It's made me interested in learning how others think and viewing the world through the lens of others and their experiences. Although my role is to help, educate, and teach my clients, I, too, become a learner and learn new things, especially in almost every birth I have ever attended. I've had beautiful births that were similar to family cookouts. I have also had serene spa-like water birth experiences. I have had silent, or almost silent, deeply spiritual births. I also have been part of an experience that felt close to nature while others were more clinical and colder. I have seen highly, highly ceremonial birth experiences, and traumatic ones too. I've seen empowering birth experiences and a little bit of everything else, I would say. Despite how much I have experienced, I keep an open mind because I understand that every birth is different and every single one is an opportunity to learn a wealth of information not only about how to respond to the experiences but also about how people work, and how to become a great source of help for others, including myself. I've learned a lot about myself in the process, too.

I often joke about something. In one of the last births I attended, the woman ended up sitting on me. We were in this birthing center, and I was going through comfort measures. I was behind her, and she was holding onto the bedpost. And I guess I was postured right behind her. And then, because I figured she felt my presence there, she went ahead and just relaxed and full-on sat on me, forcing me into a solid squat that I was not expecting.

At first, I thought, "Oh snap! I've never had a laboring woman sit on me." This lady was going through a whole contraction on my lap. I thought to myself, "I'm glad I stretched this morning because I'm doing these squats right here." It surprised everyone. The midwife rushed over to the other side of the room, grabbed the birth stool, and put it underneath me because I think none of us were expecting that. But guess what? Anything can happen in the middle of labor. And so even in that birth experience, I could say, "We squeezed hips, check. You're getting in the birthing tub, check. Counter pressure, check. Yup, that was new!"

After all these years, I'd never had someone sit on my lap while they were going through a contraction. So, I learned at that moment, "Girl, you can't forget your stretches because you do not know if your mama will sit on you today. You need to be able to hold her up, you need to be able to hold yourself up, and you need to be safe." Just when you thought you knew a little something, you learn something new. I experienced something new, and I think that it was beautiful. It was wonderful.

I've just seen so many different scenarios play out, and that's the beauty of birth work: you never know what you will witness. You don't know what's going to come up. You don't know what's going to happen and when it will happen. Stay curious, stay curious about the people you serve, authentically.

Everybody's not for you, and that is fine. It's okay if things don't play out the way you would expect them to. It will always be better for you to authentically connect with people and serve the women and their families well. It's not just a business or transaction. It is indeed an impactful experience that becomes treasured and remembered by an entire family. Unforgettable even. Sure, if you are only after the transaction, then go transactional. But that's not how I've operated, not how I view this profession. It's more than a business for me. It's deeper for me, and so I mentor and educate people from that place. I've learned that there is nothing more powerful than connection. *Connection is impact.*

About the Author

Jacquelyn Clemmons is the daughter of Wanda Simmons-Clemmons, granddaughter of Flora Simmons, great-granddaughter of Beatrice McLaughlin, the great-great-granddaughter of Naomi Leslie, and mother of three.

She is a birth and certified traditional postpartum doula/trainer, certified breastfeeding specialist, placenta specialist, doula mentor, and author. She has spent the last two decades supporting families through unmedicated, medicated, VBAC, and c-section birth experiences in the home, birth center, and hospital environments. It's been her honor to walk with families from various backgrounds and ethnicities as they journey through the joys and challenges of birth, nursing, and postpartum.

Through intuitive care, deep nourishment, and restorative support, she holds space for BIPOC families along their birth and postpartum journeys. By highlighting the energetics and spirit of birth she guides expectant families and new doulas alike.

Jacquelyn is the founding Director and CEO of Okionu Birth Foundation and OKIONU app, a non-profit organization and app that connects postpartum families of color to much-needed, culturally relevant postpartum care. Okionu Birth Foundation connects postpartum families of color to culturally relevant wrap-around support in the form of meal delivery, mental health services, and a variety of professional services. Jacquelyn's innovation and authentic leadership in the maternal health field have allowed continued transformation in the lives of families and organizations she consults for.

Mindful observation and a determination to positively impact outcomes for families of color led to her founding her startup OKIONU. A firm believer that mindfulness and authenticity are the primary pillars to not only innovating but establishing a solid company culture from the ground up, Jacquelyn has dedicated her career to empowering individuals to show up in their full glory as they build a family, pursue entrepreneurship, and their personal growth and evolution along the way.